The Joy o

19/-

P8/

THE JOY OF CANCER

Anup Kumar

Illustrations by Naved Akhtar

Rupa & Co

Published 2002 by

Rupa & Co

7/16 Ansari Road, Daryaganj
New Delhi 110 002.

Sales Centres:
Allahabad, Bangalore, Chandigarh, Chennai
Dehradun, Hyderabad, Jaipur, Kathmandu
Kolkata, Ludhiana, Mumbai, Pune

ISBN 81-7167-879-3

Typeset 11 pts. Arial by
Nikita Overseas Pvt. Ltd.
1410 Chiranjiv Tower
43 Nehru Place
New Delhi 110 019.

Printed in India by
Rekha Printers Pvt. Ltd.
A-102/1 Okhla Industrial Area
Phase-II, New Delhi 110 020.

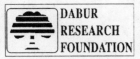

DABUR RESEARCH FOUNDATION

The book is co-sponsored by Dabur Research
Foundation, which has a R&D focus on
developing drugs and molecular diagnostics
for cancer.

To my wife
Amrita
and my daughters,
Malika and Kaveri

ACKNOWLEDGMENTS

My deepest gratitude to my wife Amrita who broke her back, literally and figuratively to keep me on my feet.

My daughters Malika and Kaveri for the dreams sacrificed without remorse or complaint.

Aruna and Saeed Naqvi, Jyoti and Satendra Nandan and Shiela and Rana Philip without whose help I wouldn't be alive today.

My mother-in-law Ivy Mohini Martin who never even knew what she did.

Poornima and Rajive Jain, Neeru and Ajai Kumar, Aruna and Sandeep Bagchee, Kamani and Brij Tankha for their unwavering love and moral support.

Amrendra Singh, Vijay Ganju, Ardeshir Dalal, Chandrashekhar Chatterji, Barun Barua, Ravindra Choudhary and Alok Punj for showing me that there is nothing like an old friend.

Feroze Gujral for the size of her heart and for holding my wife's hand when I couldn't.

Vijaylakshmi Venkatesh of the Cancer Patients Aids Association for opening doors, breaking queues, and for her friendship and good cheer.

Naved Akhtar for being able to see humour in tragedy.

Finally, those who led me through the valley of the shadow of death. Dr. D Ghosh, Dr. Sapna Nangia and Dr. HK Chaturvedi at the Batra Hospital, New Delhi; Dr. RK Deshpande and Dr. SH Advani at the Tata Memorial Hospital, Mumbai; Dr. Alok Chopra at Aashlok Hospital, New Delhi; and Dr. Navin Dang at the Medical Diagnostic Centre, New Delhi.

CONTENTS

Then a woman said, Speak to us of Joy and Sorrow.
And he answered:
Your joy is your sorrow unmasked.
And the selfsame well from which your laughter rises
was oftentimes filled with your tears.
And how else can it be?

Kahlil Gibran

FOUR MONTHS TO LIVE

January 2000. My job as vice-president of an international advertising agency was coming to an end. The company had decided to close its India operations. Advertisers all over the country were cutting back on expenditure and agencies were either in the red or shutting shop. Delayed salaries had become the norm. The writing was on the wall, yet most of us at the office were not willing to accept the inevitable. On the first working day of the new millennium, the axe fell. In a short, terse e-mail message from the CEO in New York, the marching orders were issued. We were told to close India operations by April and since the financial position of the agency was not healthy, no compensation was offered. The CEO ended by wishing everyone a happy new year.

That was how the new millennium began for me. It was not entirely unexpected but the timing was terrible. We had planned a 15-day family holiday. My wife Amrita had undertaken the renovation of her grand-uncle's 200-year-old house in Rajasthan. Repairs were in full swing. My elder daughter was getting married in a month. And suddenly, in one fell swoop, the world around me had collapsed. I had to rework my finances and cut back on expenses. The holiday was cancelled. Repairs at the old house brought to a dead halt. Most importantly, I had to start the hunt for a new job. The advertising industry was reeling under a recession and jobs simply did not exist. The few that did were better suited to someone younger than I. It was then that it dawned on me that I was on the wrong side of 50.

January ended and February was upon us. Even the remotest possibility of a job did not appear in the horizon. My daughter's wedding was two weeks away. Menus had to be finalized. Guest lists. The printing of cards. Pre-marriage celebrations. Endless visits to the tailors. More and more of my time was being devoted to the preparations. I went through that period in a haze of desperation, wondering where to cut costs. We had committed ourselves. I couldn't tell the in-laws what had happened.

It was exactly one week before the wedding that a piercing scream from the computer room shattered the silence of our household. Amrita had opened the e-mail. There, in what appeared to me as letters of gold was a message from the largest telecommunication company in the Gulf asking me to come for a job interview to Abu Dhabi. I couldn't believe my eyes.

Two days after the wedding I caught a Gulf Air flight to Abu Dhabi. From there, after a series of interviews I called home. "The nightmare's over," I said to Amrita, "start packing." She wept, the children grabbed the receiver from her and screamed congratulations into my ear. When I emerged at Delhi airport the next morning, I felt like a winner. At about the same time, I received another offer from Chennai, to head a large multinational advertising agency. Suddenly I had two jobs to choose from.

The wedding had made me bankrupt. Moreover, I had not received a salary in three months. My bills were mounting and this was the reason I finally decided to accept the Gulf job. My younger daughter had been doing quite brilliantly academically and my thought was that if I took on that job, I would be able to afford to send her abroad for further studies.

The next few weeks were spent e-mailing Abu Dhabi, back and forth, and meeting formalities, all the paperwork involved. Visas, tickets, medical check-ups, etc. Post-dated cheques that I issued all around against those mounting bills. In the frenzy, I forgot to renew my medical insurance. "Doesn't matter," I said to myself when I remembered, "who needs it now?"

April dawned. I was due to leave in two weeks. "Do hurry with those medical reports," I requested Aashlok Hospital. The following morning Dr. Alok Chopra called me in to his office and, handing me my x-ray report, told me to delay my departure. "Why?" I asked. "There's a patch on your lungs," he said. "What patch?" I said, "What do you mean?" "Could be anything," he replied, "we need to investigate." "What rubbish!" was Amrita's response when I told her. "There must be something wrong with their x-ray machine."

The tests began. First, a CT scan then a CT-guided FNAC (fine needle aspiration cytology) wherein a thin, long needle was inserted into my lungs and a minuscule portion from the patch area removed for biopsy. The results were inconclusive, so a bronchoscopy was done. Tubes fitted with laser-guided cameras were inserted into my lungs and portions of the patch and the fluid in the surrounding area were sucked out. The bronchoscopy, too, was inconclusive. It only ruled out the possibility of tuberculosis. Another FNAC was planned. The doctors persisted in taking an ominous view of that first x-ray.

Meanwhile my brother fixed an appointment for me with the much sought after Dr. R K Deshpande at the Tata Memorial Hospital in Mumbai. Though I was now desperately short of time and money I decided to go. Not in a position to afford airfare, I caught a train to Mumbai along with my newly-married daughter. It was a journey that brought back unpleasant memories. I had visited the Tata Memorial 15 years previously to discuss my mother's breast cancer with Dr. Jussawalla. My meeting with Dr. Deshpande was brief. He looked at all my papers and reports and asked me to get another FNAC done at the Breach Candy Hospital. He would not hazard a guess as to whether the patch was malignant or benign but he did insist that I undergo the procedure for a complete diagnosis. "We need to take things step by step Mr Kumar," he said in the face of my growing impatience.

The following morning the thin, long needle was once again plunged deep into my lungs. Early the next day, as the doors of the lab were being opened, my daughter and I arrived at the Metropolis Laboratory for the biopsy result. The meeting with the doctor there did not last more than five minutes. Five minutes in which I realized that my life would never be the same again. "Mr. Kumar," she said, "your biopsy results show malignancy. Poorly differentiated adenocarcinoma. You should meet Dr. Deshpande. He will advise you on your next course of treatment."

Perhaps I should have been prepared. Right from the beginning the doctors had warned me that because I had been a heavy smoker for over 35 years the chances of malignancy were high. All considered, I found myself hoping against hope that there was some error of judgment in the biopsy report. That my FNAC sample had been interchanged with another. Or the laboratory had received samples from two patients bearing the same name! Unfortunately that was not to be. I had to accept the truth with as much dignity and grace as possible.

Dr. Deshpande was reassuring. He said the patch was small, that the effected portion of my lungs needed to be surgically removed and that in about four to six weeks I would be on my feet. However, a complete body scan had to be conducted before surgery could commence. I heard my daughter call home from a nearby phone. "Please catch the first available flight," I heard her say to my wife. "And bring Rs 2 lakh with you." I knew my wife had no more than Rs 400 in her cupboard. And there had been nothing in the bank for a long time. I stared at the walls helplessly. Things were moving beyond my control.

The following day was hectic. Blood tests. Ultrasounds. CT scans. Bone scans. ECG. Echo cardiography. And more. It was while I was waiting my turn for the bone scan that I had my first glimpse of a cancer ward. It was a grim sight, with a number of people without hair, some with caps, some wearing scarves. Most had an oddly blank expression on their faces as if they had been sitting in the same position for years. As if they had lost control of their destiny. A few were distinctly uncomfortable, perhaps in pain. Which one of them was I going to become?

By the evening I had been admitted into Breach Candy hospital for the surgery. Lying in bed I looked at the turgid brown waves lashing against the black rocks that fringed the sea face of the hospital. For the first time in two weeks the enormity of what lay ahead dawned on me. I was alone with my thoughts. My daughter had returned to Delhi, Amrita had arrived along with a friend and they were busy collecting all my reports from the various departments. Lost in my own thoughts and as a result of a long and tiring day, I must have drifted into sleep.

I awoke to a flurry of activity in my room. Doctors and

nurses were talking in hushed tones. From the corner of my eye, I could see Amrita staring fixedly at the sea. She wouldn't turn around. Then Dr. Deshpande walked in and said that some "small" doubt had surfaced in the bone scan results, which needed to be confirmed through a MRI examination. "Let's take it step by step," he said once more.

At 9 pm I was wheeled into a dimly lit room that was dominated by a huge canon-shaped machine. After I lay down, a small switch was placed in my hand and I was told that I could press the button in case I panicked. The roof was barely 10-15 cm from the tip of my nose. It was a nightmare. In the one and a half hours that I lay trapped the only thing that stopped me from pressing the button was the thought that this horrific test would have to then begin all over again.

Results came by morning. The grim expression on Dr. Deshpande's face as he walked into my room told me all. Surgery would be futile. The cancer had spread to the bones. "Your cancer has reached Stage Four, I'm afraid," he said. "How many stages are there?" my wife asked hesitantly. Dr. Deshpande looked away as he answered. "Four," he said. I saw my wife's face not change expression. I saw her swallow.

For me, the bed, the floor, everything seemed to have suddenly disappeared from under me. Dr. Deshpande left saying that he would fix an appointment for me with his colleague, Dr. Advani at the Tata Memorial. So a short while later I checked out of Breach Candy, physically whole but stunned. At the Tata Memorial, Dr. Advani prepared a chemotherapy protocol that he said could be administered in Delhi. His assessment of my situation was summed up in these words, "Mr Kumar, if you don't respond to the chemotherapy treatment, you have only about four months to live."

Back home and armed with that protocol, I visited all the major cancer hospitals. The Rajiv Gandhi Institute was too far away, so was Dharamshila. The All India Institute of Medical Sciences, practically at my doorstep, was too crowded. I finally decided on Batra Hospital.

The day before chemotherapy was to begin, the story was once again turned on its head. After re-examining my reports and films, the doctors at Batra Hospital came to the conclusion that surgery was a better option. More tests were conducted to confirm their diagnosis. I even took a second opinion from the Tumor Board at the Rajiv Gandhi Hospital. So chemotherapy was suddenly cancelled, the drugs returned, and I found myself waiting to be operated upon for the second time. I had no idea that a cancer diagnosis could be so complicated.

The following day a 35 cm gash was made across my chest, some ribs removed, but in the end my lung stayed exactly where it was because the surgeon discovered to his shock that the cancer had spread right through the pleura. Multiple small deposits all over the upper and middle lobe of the right lung were seen. None of this had shown up in any test. I was stapled up and wheeled into the ICU. The whole exercise had been a huge waste and yet I would have to go through the various stages of post-operative recovery. Worse, I had to pay the exorbitant fee for the operation despite the fact that I had nothing but a massive scar to show for it. Worse yet, I was now too weak for chemotherapy and precious time had been lost.

One of the doctors who had been present at the operation told Amrita unofficially that I shouldn't be made to go through chemotherapy at all. It was too late, he said. By the looks of my insides I had only four to five months to live. I should be allowed to die peacefully. Chemotherapy would torment me, he said, and extend my life by only another two months at most. Chances of cure were as low as 10%. It was a horrifying prognosis. Family and friends urged me to try ayurvedic or homeopathic medicine, or even Tibetan. While I was still recovering from the post-operative trauma my daughter raced off to Dharamsala to meet the famous Dr. Yeshi Donden. A niece meanwhile went to Dehradun to meet a world-renowned homeopath.

I was willing to experiment with alternative medicine but finally I settled for chemotherapy. Statistics didn't support the decision but I had made up my mind to blast those statistics. I simply wasn't willing to die. Even on the chemotherapy protocol there were differences of opinion. The aggressive 3-drug protocol prescribed by Dr. Advani was reduced to two drugs, Taxotere and Cisplatin. I studied carefully all the possible side effects of these drugs. Whatever I read frightened me. It seemed that a survey once conducted amongst 79 Canadian oncologists indicated that all of them would encourage their patients to go in for chemotherapy but only 58 per cent would agree to chemotherapy if they themselves had lung cancer, and *81 per cent would not allow Cisplatin to be administered under any circumstances!* Apparently the side effects of Cisplatin were horrendous. But in my case, Cisplatin it was. The doctors said it was the only chance I had, however small.

Chemotherapy began in June. For six months I was bombed out of my senses. Within a few days I lost my hair. The nausea and vomiting, and the intermittent constipation and diarrhea, dehydrated me completely. I began losing weight and my blood count dropped to alarmingly low levels. I became weak and often needed support to walk around the house. As the chemotherapy progressed, the cumulative effects   became worse. Both arms were daily injected with needles, either to draw blood samples or to receive either glucose or a blood transfusion, and of course, the chemotherapy drugs. With the continuous puncturing, my veins collapsed. So I was once again wheeled into the operation theatre. Under local anesthesia, a chemo-port was inserted under my left shoulder and connected to the main artery leading to the heart. At times my immunity plunged to dangerously low levels and I had to be isolated. Those who entered my room had to leave their shoes outside the door and wear a protective mask. Communicate with me from a distance to avoid passing on infection. I would barely spend a few days at home before being rushed back to hospital on account of one emergency or another. The house itself began to look like a mini nursing home. For a period I took 27 tablets a day, apart from daily injections.

By the end of the fourth cycle, some damage to my hearing was noticed. I was also suffering from peripheral neuropathy, a condition that meant that my lower limbs had been adversely affected by the drugs, resulting in wobbly knees whenever I stood or walked. I was given electric shocks and the electro-physiological study showed damage that only time could possibly heal. At the same time I developed hypotension that meant that my blood pressure readings varied depending on whether I was lying down, sitting or standing. Again and again I was rushed to hospital, and kept under observation of cardiologists and other specialists. A point came when I became too weak to even understand what was going on. The chemo-port was working overtime with intravenous fluids, antibiotic injections and blood transfusions. Towards the end new drugs were administered to reduce the side effects of the treatment.

All this while my x-ray and CT scan results were indicating that I was making progress. After the first set of results, the chemotherapy protocol was made even more aggressive. The maximum permissible dosage of the two drugs was being administered and the oncologists were beginning to see signs of total cure. But at the same time the side effects of the treatment were taking their toll. The last time I left the hospital it was on a wheel chair. I could hardly hold my head up. But I was alive. And the treacherous patch in my lungs was gone.

Most of this book was written during those horrifying six months, in between bouts of nausea and all the other side effects of chemotherapy. It is largely based on my own experiences but also on conversations with other cancer patients and their families. The main part enumerates a seven-point battle plan that saw me through the worst days of my life. I am hoping it will see you through yours.

Anup Kumar
New Delhi
January 2002

7-POINT BATTLE PLAN

But if the flame dies out,
the world becomes a dark and frightening place.
We lose both our way
and the one way to find a way.
Bani Shorter in *How Does it Really Feel?*

BATTLE PLAN 1
ACCEPTING YOUR CANCER

I n a short period of less than two weeks my life had taken an about turn. Several about turns. Instead of leaving for Abu Dhabi, I had walked through many corridors of many hospitals. I was educated, unemployed and my lungs were riddled with cancer. I had been turned away from a lobectomy in which a part of my right lung would have been removed. Surgery that had been confirmed only twenty-four hours previously. Surgery that was cancelled minutes before it was to begin. Surgery for which I had spent twenty-four hours preparing my mind, body and soul to accept.

Amrita and I drove in silence through the crowded streets of Mumbai. In a short span of time her life, too, had changed dramatically. Nothing that I could have said would have mattered. Nothing that she could have said would have helped. As we entered the premises of the Tata Memorial Hospital, uppermost in my mind was, What had I done to deserve this?

Yes. What indeed had I done to deserve this? I was confronted with the inevitable 'Why *me*' question. What was the difference between me and the man across the street? Me and the rest of the world? And, conversely, what was so special about me that *my* lungs could not be afflicted with cancer cells? And, would I have wished that my best friend had cancer instead of me? Or any of my near and dear ones? Or my worst enemy even? No. I was the chosen one. Did I have it in me to save myself from cancer? Not in the medical sense but every other way that could support medical treatment? What changes was I to anticipate in my life? What changes would I be able to cope with?

In retrospect, there is a good side to being confronted with a final diagnosis, howsoever painful that diagnosis might be. Until then, I had taken each day and each test result as it came with a mixture of bewilderment, disbelief, despair and hope. After being torn apart in this manner, there was an odd comfort in finally knowing the truth. At least I knew where I stood.

In the following days I spoke to my body. Tenderly, lovingly, gently. I wanted each part of my being to be ready for the long struggle that lay ahead. For the parts that were not yet affected, I had to ensure that there was no way that the cancer cells could enter and take control. I began to realize that only I had the power to control my body. My body was *me*. Together we had to be prepared.

It might seem like a strange way to look at a cancer diagnosis, but the truth is that your body *is* you, healthy or not, and going outside yourself to look upon that body from a distance, in disdain, or in fear, is the worst thing you can do. In my mind I said a short prayer thanking God for *our* first victory. And from that moment in time there was no looking back in anger. No turning around to see my life crumble before me. I was a cancer patient and there was nothing in the world that could alter that fact. No amount of rage or grief could change things around.

It was then that I realized that the treatment, control or cure, were as much in my hands as they were in the hands of the doctors. I had to learn to navigate my ship in a manner that was totally alien to me. I had to change the way I saw and did most things in my life. I could not worry about trivial things like being unemployed. These things would change automatically as and when it was time for them to change. I was fighting a war against cancer. A war of many battles deep inside my own territory. In a terrain that I was not totally familiar with. It was a war that I could not afford to lose.

In a short span of time, I changed dramatically. In my attitude towards everything and everyone who was near and dear to me. I was preparing to live my life with a single-minded purpose. For the next six to eight months. Or much longer, if I survived beyond that period. To the doctors, statistics were what mattered. To them I was a Stage Four cancer patient. In other words, I was as good as dead. I had no option but to blast those statistics.

The first stage of the treatment begins with acceptance. Not hesitant acceptance but total acceptance. Don't expect doctors to help you do this, they have far too much else to deal with, but they do agree that when a patient is cured, it is because *both* mind and body were in a state of acceptance. You cannot just wish cancer away. No amount of remorse or prayers can revert a medical diagnosis. And the sooner this harsh reality is accepted, the sooner you can move towards coping with cancer.

Getting into the 'Why *me*?' syndrome is lethal. Often the 'Why *me*?' is compounded by 'Why *now*?' And that makes acceptance even more difficult. Moreover, you will soon find yourself surrounded by well-meaning friends and relatives who begin to talk the same language. To avoid such an unhappy state of affairs, you, the patient, must take charge.

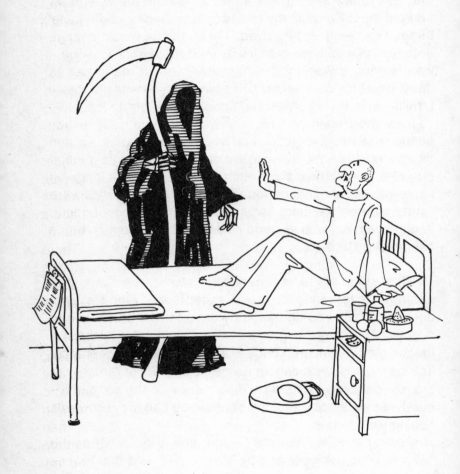

"Wait a minute! I want a second opinion."

Remember always, how you communicate with the world is the way the world will communicate with you. And your communication must start from *within*. How can you reject a part of your own being? Those bad cells are an integral part of you. Rejecting them would be like rejecting yourself. And the more you turn away from the truth, the more the malignancy of the disease begins to gain the upper hand. Try thinking of your cancer as an unwelcome guest. You might wish it would go away soon, but don't slam the door in its face. It doesn't work.

Don't delay the acceptance stage because with cancer there is very little time to lose. You need time to build your army for battle. Each day wasted is an opportunity for the cells to gain advantage. If you are completely ignorant about cancer, and this is causing nameless fears in you, read all you can about the disease at this stage, or surf the net. There are huge amounts of information available today. Knowledge reduces fear. There are innumerable horrifying myths about cancer that need to be dispelled and learning the truth about the disease is the way to do it.

I still remember that first night after the final diagnosis, wondering how to accept what had happened to me. I couldn't sleep. I felt deeply alone. Rather than wake up my wife who had had a grueling day, I decided to have a serious chat with my lungs. I reasoned with the cancer cells. I asked for their forgiveness. I asked them to be good friends with me. I made peace with them. In the morning when I described my experience to Amrita, she looked at me in alarm. She thought I was losing my mind. But drastic circumstances call for drastic methods. It takes time for others to understand the state of mind of a cancer patient.

I spent the next few days re-living my life. My earliest memories were of carefree days at St. Columba's School. Summer holidays spent with my maternal grandmother who did not survive cancer herself. As also my mother. I recalled the happy moments we spent together. The college years. The first cigarette I smoked. The circumstances of my marriage. Bringing up the children. Our holidays together as a family. My various jobs. So when was it decided that as soon as I turned 50, I would become a cancer patient? Had I the power to change my karma? And along with it, my mother's karma? Or my grandmother's karma? Only when I succeeded in doing so, my guruji explained to me, would members of the generations to follow be rid of the disease. This may or may not appeal to many cancer patients but as a philosophy it brought me infinite comfort.

What is karma? In simple terms it represents the destiny created for oneself, based on the laws of cause and effect. The effects we experience in the present are the inevitable results of causes that we have created in the past, either in this lifetime or over many previous lifetimes. And similarly, the causes we create now will determine the nature of the future we will either enjoy or suffer. Karma means action and refers to the fact that every action leads to a future action, in an unbroken chain throughout eternity. We create our own karma. Through our thoughts, our words, our deeds, and all of these in turn express our karma. Karma is not an external or outside force but rather the effects of causes of the past, that continue to have a profound influence on present actions. Some of the effects of these causes may be latent for years, for many lifetimes, while some, which may have already manifested themselves, could have resulted in one's present condition. If we want to understand the causes made in the past, we should look at the effects as they appear in the present. And to know what results will occur in the future, we need to analyze and look at the causes that are being formed now. Clearly the concept of karma teaches us that no one is responsible for our lives except we ourselves. Karma means that everything we suffer, everything we enjoy, is the result of our own actions, without any exception. And even the changing of our own karma, therefore, is in our own hands. Rather than forever worry about whether we are making good or bad causes, we should purify our inner spirit that motivates our various actions.

So I thought about ways to change my karma. There was an urgent need to remove any hatred for the cancer cells inside my lungs, since intense hatred leads to the accumulation of evil karma. Even when the resentment is directed within oneself, a form of evil karma gets activated. As this resentment translates into rage, a stronger evil karma gets created.

Some people say that cancer is self-imposed, often caused by deep-rooted resentment held for a long period of time until it literally starts eating away at the body. When, where and how the process begins is difficult to fathom. It could go back to one's childhood. A hurt that remained unexpressed for a long period of time, never really forgotten. An event with deep-rooted consequences that victimize you all the subsequent years of your life. Making it difficult sometimes for a person to sustain long term, meaningful relationships. Life is visualized as a series of disappointments for which *others,* and not oneself, are to blame. And within all these numerous interconnected series of past events, cancer could creep into the system. Once detected, it is important to develop a positive attitude to everything around. Learn to love again. Accept the self. These are the first steps of the healing process. Sustaining these feelings and attitudes during the treatment is the more difficult part in the fight against cancer. And that is where most battles are won, or lost.

In the beginning, all this made sense. I re-lived my childhood to understand when and where things went wrong. When was it that I had allowed cancer to creep into my system? What was it about me that had weakened my defenses, allowed those cells to go mad? If I was to regain my health, then I had to face the fact that I alone was responsible for my cancer. And therefore, only I had the power to get rid of that cancer. I had to draw upon all my reserves, all my inner strength, to make my body and mind healthy once again. I would win each battle with a new approach and style that would confuse the cancer cells themselves. The random laws that governed them. Create a new mind-body continuum. That was the task at hand. Nothing else mattered. My unemployment. My broken commitments.

Deep introspection. Long moments of solitude. Till I had succeeded in re-living 50 years of my life. Till I had found the answers to how and when and why I had become a cancer patient. And it was then that I was able to finalize my battle plan. Total acceptance to start with, backed by a positive attitude and the will to lead from the front by participating in the treatment at all times. Easier said than done. It was at this stage that I remembered my mother's treatment, and that it would be a long haul. Somehow I just had to minimize the pain and the suffering.

Memories of my grandmother's fight against cancer and also my own mother's experiences with cancer haunted me. My grandmother was 74 years old when it happened. Short, frail, extremely religious and made of sterner stuff than I. Chemotherapy at her time was not an accepted form of cancer treatment. She was advised surgery and a mastectomy was performed at the Kanpur Medical College where her son was a professor in anesthesiology. She was then moved to Delhi and radiation was used to bring her cancer under control. However, though she had an extremely positive attitude throughout, her age and her frail health did not allow her to cope with the treatment. She suffered a great deal, and was given morphine injections to help her bear the pain towards the end. Her son, my uncle, a Major in the Indian Army, told me later that she had often pleaded with him to help her end her life. I had moved to Bombay by then. It was there that I had received a black-bordered postcard informing me that my grandmother had passed away. It was the first death that affected me deeply. Even today, some 26 years later, I remember my grandmother as someone who was full of love, courage and unselfish caring. I remember her fondness for her grandchildren and the many summers that we spent at her palatial home in Lucknow. Sleeping in the garden under a huge mango tree. Stealing raw mangoes at night when she was fast asleep. Cancer had taken her away from me. And now it was in my mind and body, inside my lungs. I was carrying the family burden of cancer. I was the new flag bearer. And I had to win the war that had begun so many years ago.

In my mother's case, the experiences were vastly different. When I carried her reports to the Tata Memorial for a second opinion, I was unaware that I would repeat that terrible journey for myself years later. She underwent a mastectomy at the All India Institute of Medical Sciences, New Delhi. Subsequently, radiotherapy was administered since she was unable to cope with the side effects of chemotherapy. She did manage, however, to take the chemotherapy drugs in the form of pills, which obviously weren't as efficacious. I remember her nausea, her lack of appetite, her pain, her suffering, her weakness, and all the other side effects of the treatment as if it were only yesterday. I pictured myself in her place and wondered whether I would be able to cope with the treatment if I had to go through what she went through. Would I be able to sustain my inner strength till the end? And at what cost would victory be achieved? All sorts of fears and anxieties flashed through my mind. Her weakness, her low blood counts and immunity levels, all seemed to suddenly appear as fresh and real as when they had happened over 15 years ago. I could now identify with her symptoms much better. My mother and I were in the same boat except that she was no longer there in person. How wonderful it would have been if she were by my bedside, advising me on how to overcome pain. I mourned her loss all over again. In the last six to seven years of her life, she seemed to have given up on her fight. She was not able to cope any more. Could I have done more to help her? On the sad morning when she left the world, a deep chill descended upon me. At her funeral I sat close to the burning pyre until the heat of its flames rising in the sky became unbearable. And as I sat and stared at her body being turned to ash, somewhere deep down I had a premonition that I was never able to put my finger on. Was this what that premonition was about? Was my mother trying to tell me something?

Somehow I had to alter that karma. Ensure not only that cancer was forever banished from my system but from my children's future, their children's future. Perhaps this sounds pompous, and moreover, on a scientific plain none of this makes sense, but for me the moment of reckoning had arrived. Changing my karma was essential. I have no logical explanation for this thought process. Perhaps it arose from the heart of a father, full of fear for what he might pass on to his children. It was *my* way of coping, of creating some sense out of chaos.

Once you've accepted the fact that you have cancer, you're in the happy position of being able to notice its benefits. So many emerged in my life, which is why I called this book *The Joy of Cancer*. Amrita disapproved. So did my daughters. "Aren't you stretching things a bit?" they said. So I made up my mind to list those benefits, explain what I was talking about. And thinking about these benefits helped me towards a greater acceptance of the disease. Especially during the times when I was suffering the side effects of chemotherapy.

First, the air in the house changed drastically for the better. There used to be a pall of nicotine smoke hanging over it. I had been a heavy smoker all my adult life. 30 to 40 cigarettes a day for over 35 years. Nearly 500,000 cigarettes, I estimated. The children had always disliked my smoking. Like all smokers I had made brave but unsuccessful attempts to give up. These attempts lasted all of five to seven days and then sure enough, back I was to this repulsive habit. The house had a stale smell always. Filthy ashtrays. The smell had permeated the fabric of the house, the curtains, the sofas, my hair, my skin. It was the same case with my office. I don't know how many passive smokers I must have initiated. Addicts are shameless and selfish because it was only when I was told I had lung cancer did the desire for tobacco disappear. I had no withdrawal symptoms either. Never will a cigarette cross my lips again. I am beginning to feel healthier. My energy levels have increased. "Have I not benefited?" I asked my daughters. So have they, in fact, since they are no longer passive smokers.

Second, I learned who my friends are. It's a hugely comfortable feeling. We all go through life wondering whether we've invested our energies and our affections in the right people. Now I know. The line between those who care and those who don't is clearly drawn when you're in trouble. As the news that I had cancer spread among friends and family, I was flooded with telephone calls, visitors and 'get well soon' messages. They came from all corners of the world, old college friends whom I had very little to do with in decades. The first surprise was that I knew so many people, had so many well-wishers. They gave me words of encouragement. They boosted my spirits. They helped me overcome my initial fears. They gave me advice from the experiences of friends and relatives. They brought books for me to read. Took the trouble even, to order some titles on the internet. Soon I had one of the largest libraries on the subject. They downloaded relevant extracts from the internet and gave me printouts. They held my hand in hospital. They comforted Amrita and my daughters. The result: I suddenly felt wanted. I suddenly had a strong desire to win the war against cancer. It strengthened my resolve. Above all, it created bonds that I hadn't succeeded in creating all my life.

Third, I was freed from the vicious cycle of workaholism. Often I had worked late into the night either at home or at office. Family holidays were not on my agenda. Amrita was angry, the children were repeatedly disappointed when plans to leave town were cancelled. It had become so bad that nobody even suggested a holiday anymore. I myself was perpetually irritable and exhausted. Initially, I was terrified when I realized I had no office to go to anymore. And then gradually, as I began to introspect, to read, to play bridge again (a past passion) and surf the internet, I became a more 'normal' and laid-back person. As a result, I found my lost family. Despite the cancer, the sounds of laughter and conversation could be heard in my home again. I began to look at life with a new perspective. My identity was no longer in my suit, my tie, and my polished shoes. I was free. It was a new life. It was different. It was what I had dreamed of for a long time and not known how to achieve.

As time elapsed, I also became spiritual. I found solace and peace in Buddhist chanting and meditation. On some days, I could spend hours observing time pass by. Stare through my window and observe the marvels of nature. The different shades of green on the leaves outside. Hear the birds chirp. Listen to the distant barking of stray dogs. The sound of an occasional aircraft that flew overhead. Simple things began to give me joy. Things that I had not noticed in years. It was ironical that in the face of death, I began, for the first time, to really live.

Of course the odds were against me but it is important to accept both the bad *and* the good. The human soul at peace is strong ammunition against malignant cells.

Can cancer differentiate between people? How is it that some people survive the disease and others don't? Some of it has to do with tension. Cancer, or any other illness for that matter, is reason enough to increase tension in your life. As a cancer patient, you can do without tension and negative feelings. Once you are aware, once you have accepted the truth, you are on the road to health. Medical advice and treatment is only half the fight. The balance is in your own hands.

You're the general. It's your body, your health, your money. Everyone else is hired help.

Anne E. Frahm in *Cancer Battle Plan*

BATTLE PLAN 2
CHOOSING YOUR TREATMENT
AND YOUR DOCTORS

A cancer diagnosis can be devastating. It can bring about a wide variety of emotions and reactions, including fear, shock, anger, disbelief and panic. Initially the fact that you are singled out as a cancer patient is difficult to comprehend. You feel that your body, or at least some part of it, has let you down. One moment life is normal and the next everything has changed. Instead of meetings at offices there are endless trips to hospitals. Innumerable restrictions get imposed on you. The future too does not appear so bright. The days are never the same again. Priorities have to be redefined. There is little time to be lost. There is information to be gathered, things to be done, and decisions to be made. Life is turned upside down.

I was no different. The words "Mr Kumar, you have lung cancer" still reverberate in my memory. Sing a tune that will never be forgotten. After I heard those words, things moved fast, mostly beyond my control, and somewhere in the midst of it all, shock, anger and disbelief receded in the distant background. It dawned on me that the situation in my lungs was no different to what it was before the diagnosis. The only difference being that earlier I had no inkling of the havoc that was being created in my right lung. Now I was that much wiser.

A considerable amount of background research on alternative treatment therapies and introspection was all that I could show for the time that had whizzed past. I had not yet entered the treatment mode. Mine was a fast-growing variety of lung cancer. I knew there was little time to be lost. The war had to be waged fast. It would have to be fought on many fronts, with a judicious mix of both conventional and psychological warfare. The battleground was known. The enemy was deeply entrenched in a small, one-inch diameter patch in my right lung. Additional territory had come under enemy control, in the pleura region. The war would be a long drawn-out affair. Many battles would be fought. Some would be won and others lost. I had to marshal my troops immediately.

The delay in treatment had given me sufficient time to develop my own battle plan. Sufficient knowledge had been acquired, and proper sifting of the information collected was essential. Chemotherapy would be the ace up my sleeve, supported in good measure by a few options in alternative therapies. I had done the rounds of clinics earlier. Clinics run by homeopaths, vaids, naturopaths, ayurveds, reiki healers, faith healers, Tibetan medicine practitioners and many more. They all had more or less the same thing to say. "Chemotherapy is expensive and offers no guarantee of cure or control. Besides, it has a whole lot of undesirable side effects. Have trust in us and we assure you of a complete cure."

The final decision was always left to me. And I had neither complete knowledge nor the expertise to choose the best course of action. The more people I spoke to, both in the medical profession and among cancer patients, the more confused I became. The response in the end was always "the decision is yours". Little knowledge is supposed to be a dangerous thing. To me it appeared that the more knowledge I gained the more difficult it became to make the right decision.

The vaid, without even examining me or asking details about my case, said that tulsi leaves, gangajal and a young cow's urine consumed twice every day were the perfect cure for cancer. The tulsi plant was acquired and two jars of the yellow liquid lay in my room for a couple of days. However in the end, I could not bring myself to drink it.

My elder daughter visited Dr. Yeshi Donden at Dharamshala, the former advisor to the Dalai Lama. As per his request, she had taken with her an early morning sample of my urine. Apparently when my case was put in front of him, he examined my urine sample against the sunlight, and shaking the bottle, said "Your father has lung cancer." My daughter was stunned. How could a urine sample seen against sunlight confirm the nature of the disease? She returned with three different medicines. I started the course immediately, but gave it up later since a number of people told me that Tibetan medicine was not particularly known for lung cancer cure. Right or wrong, I was not sure. My faith in this form of treatment was high, especially after the way the diagnosis was made. After a few weeks of taking the medication as prescribed, I decided to stop because I was also told it would clash terribly with chemotherapy. Perhaps I could return to it at a later stage, I thought.

The homeopath, on the other hand, listened patiently to my story. He then consulted two large books on homeopathy. After careful study, he disappeared inside his clinic, returning with two envelopes, each containing a phial of pills. "Start with these and come back to me if any fresh symptoms emerge," he said triumphantly. Adding as I was leaving, "Trust me and my medication and your cancer will be gone in no time." I went home elated. From the next day onwards, I religiously followed his advice both in terms of the diet and the medication. No fresh symptoms arose. Then I read an article that confirmed my earlier doubts about the efficacy of homeopathic medication for advanced stages of lung cancer. I gradually lost interest and never went back to the homeopath for further advice. Till today I am not sure whether my decision was right or wrong.

The naturopath started by examining the position of the planets in my life using her computer and concluded that two planets were not in the correct position. This had resulted in my present health problem. Both planets were expected to shift from their position to a more favourable position by the middle of July when my health would begin to improve. In the meantime she would advise me as to what needed to be done to reduce the effects of the unfavourable position of the planets. And also, subsequently, what I would have to do to get rid of the cancer. This included a strict diet regimen, wearing of specific colours on specific days, and so on. I would have to follow her advice strictly and the cancer would disappear in no time. Somehow I was not convinced by her faith and decided that I would not go back to her for further consultations.

The faith healer was a similar story. Drink three cups of light tea made from green tea leaves, some seeds (I don't remember their names now) and ginger, along with garlic. At the same time, my family and I were supposed to pray three to four times a day. A special prayer was given to me for this purpose. While she gave me instances of when and where the treatment had worked, I personally was not convinced. Another faith healer that I visited tossed a coin each time he answered my questions, wanted to make my janampatri and said he would perform some special rites at his temple in Mumbai. Even though he talked about a number of successful cases, I was far from convinced.

I had come across many interesting stories related to ayurvedic medicine. Many patients, some friends, some friends of friends, had taken ayurvedic medicine along with chemotherapy, and had shown remarkable progress. Whoever we spoke to had something positive to say. Each one we spoke to swore by his or her ayurved. From Raigarh to Varanasi. From Dehradun to Trivandrum. From Jaipur to Delhi. Ayurveds who had successfully treated cancer patients seemed to be everywhere, each more famous and renowned than the other. Some even mentioned cases that they had treated which had been written off by the Sloane Kettering Memorial Hospital in New York. Initially, the ayurvedic treatment appeared extremely promising, with the added benefit of there being no known side effects to this form of medication. The problem was more to do with the choice of ayurved, since each one seemed to have impeccable credentials. Finally I decided to meet a renowned New Delhi ayurved. I took his medicine for about two months, stopping it only when I had his prescribed drugs analyzed at a laboratory. To my horror, the drugs were nothing but a strong dose of steroids.

I could continue with such stories endlessly. In no way should my experience or some of the examples cited earlier be taken as complete truths. Each patient must decide for himself or herself. The advice given to me by Dr. Alok Chopra of Aashlok Hospital, who has studied and analyzed more than fifty forms of alternative medicine and is setting up a clinic for various disciplines in the field of medicine, was most valuable. In his words: "Every form of alternative medicine has its benefits. The patient has to be convinced that a particular form will do him or her good for any kind of medication to be effective. Even modern medicine works on the same principle. And ideally, to derive the best results, the patient must live his or her life as per the demands of that particular form of medication. For instance, to get the best results from Tibetan or ayurvedic medicine, the patient must reorganize his or her life according to the Tibetan or Vedic way of life."

Back to where I started. Even after nearly eight weeks and an unsuccessful surgery to show for it, the final decision on the course of my treatment was left to me. Time was running out. As a student of science and having always trusted modern allopathic medication, even for minor fever and coughs and colds all my life, I decided to start with chemotherapy and support it with ayurvedic treatment and reiki healing. Besides, Dr. Chopra had confirmed that only modern medicine had records to confirm the success rates in cancer treatment. All other forms of alternative medicine did not maintain proper records and therefore their results could not be validated.

I felt elated. Finalizing the treatment was another major step towards ultimate victory. The choice of hospital and the team of doctors was the decision left to be made. Delhi, like most other major Indian cities, offers a large number of hospitals and even private nursing homes for cancer treatment. The distance factor from my residence was an important consideration in the choice of the hospital. Apart from the number of trips that would be necessary for the chemotherapy delivery, there would be an equal number, if not many more, that would be essential for the various tests like x-rays, CT scans, bone scans, etc. Most oncologists prefer that these tests be conducted at the same hospital where the chemotherapy is being administered for ease of internal consultation. Also, chemotherapy treatment needs a constant monitoring of various critical parameters of the blood. The latter, however, can also be conducted at any reliable pathological laboratory. Lastly, check-ups and consultations are essential when the side effects of the chemotherapy become unmanageable. At times even hospitalization is necessary. Proximity therefore is critical. The Rajiv Gandhi Cancer Hospital was too far from where we lived. The All India Medical Institute, though nearby, was too crowded. Apollo Hospital and Dharamshila Cancer Institute were also ruled out because of the distance factor. Private nursing homes like Aashlok did not have all the support and test facilities that would be necessary. Batra Hospital for me was the most convenient.

Another aspect that is critical to choosing a hospital is your own comfort level with the team of doctors who will work with you on your treatment. It is not just enough to talk to the doctors. Nor is it enough to understand what they have to say. You must also talk to their patients. Share their experiences. How much confidence do the doctors inspire? Not just the senior consultants, but also the junior doctors, the nurses and other support staff right down to even the billing department. How long can the togetherness be sustained? There are bound to be differences in opinions as your battle plan unfolds. In my experience, I found that the 'me doctor, you patient' formula did not work. Partnership is the key. Though the doctors might know much more than you do about medicine, it's *your* life that you are putting in their hands. You have a right to know all the whys and the wherefores. What is being done to you and why. To analyze what is being prescribed. The 'doctor is the boss' syndrome just does not work with cancer.

In Indian hospitals, the crowd factor is equally important. I refer to the crowd factor since this effects the patient as well as the large number of people who usually accompany the patient. When Amrita and I visited the All India Medical Institute, the cancer wing was been renovated and expanded. The out-patients department comprised a medium-sized room with five or six beds with little or no privacy. And in this cramped space, I noticed that chemotherapy was being administered to all patients. Getting a private room was next to impossible. This was extremely important for me since one of my chemotherapy drugs required an overnight stay at the hospital, the administration needing about five to six hours of hydration before and after the drug was administered. Most of the other hospitals that we visited had small, private cubicles in the out-patients department for chemotherapy delivery. This, we concluded, would be a definite advantage.

Batra Hospital which we finally decided on became like my second home. At times there was a long wait for my turn. I utilized these occasions to talk to my fellow patients. Find out more about cancer. Learn from their experiences. Their strategies to win the war. Exchange notes. Share feelings of anguish. Of hope.

Most large hospitals in major Indian cities are fully equipped with all facilities essential for cancer treatment. This not only includes the various departments necessary to monitor progress, but also others that are essential to analyze any side effects. The same may not be true of the smaller nursing homes. Cancer treatment requires a wide variety of services. I realized this only later. Not just the routine imaging departments but, as a cumulative result of the chemotherapy

I had to undergo tests at the audio laboratory, the clinical neurophysiology laboratory as also some complicated cardiac tests. Such facilities are only available at large hospitals and for this reason the smaller nursing homes do not make sense. Specialists are essential who could be called upon for their expert opinion as and when complications arise.

It is important to also conduct a check on hospital costs and charges. Cancer is a rich man's disease. During my numerous trips to hospital I met patients and their families from all sections of society. The son who had to sell his farm to meet the expenses of his father's cancer. Families that had gone deep in debt in their war against cancer. We were no different. While very little can be done in terms of the high cost of chemotherapy drugs, hospital charges can differ. Doctor's fees. Room costs for overnight stay. Numerous tests that have to be conducted. All these add up to large sums of money.

I was stunned to hear that one of my chemotherapy drugs would cost me well over Rs 1 lakh each time. And that there were innumerable other expenses as well. The unending hospital bills. Medication to fight and control the side effects. Repeated tests to monitor the progress of the treatment. Over a period of only six months, my treatment cost me approximately Rs 12 lakh. Amrita and I did not have that kind of money. She had decided to take this burden off my shoulders. It was only much later that I learned that all the valuables we possessed had been sold. All the jewelry she owned, including her wedding ring. She borrowed large sums from two of her sisters and from friends. Only I know what it must have cost her, how she would have suffered. But the subject of funds for my treatment and our increasing debt was never discussed. She maintained a stoic silence. As I watched the money flow from her hands like water from the Ganga I became more and more determined to win.

As far as attitudes towards doctors go, you must remember that doctors are as human as you are. Uppermost in their minds is your well-being and recovery. Yet being human, they are as fallible as you are. They too can make mistakes. Like my not-so-necessary surgery. Today's medical delivery system, especially in large and busy hospitals, allows less and less time for doctors to spend with their patients. Yet the amount of time spent is not significant, as is the quality of time that is shared. Traditionally the doctor's role has been restricted to diagnosing the patient's disease and then treating it. This is gradually changing as the information revolution is making patients more and more aware of their health status. And doctors are beginning to be more sensitive to their patients' needs.

On your part, you must understand how valuable time is for a doctor. He almost always has patients in queue. From the very first visit, you must carefully listen to the advice offered and be ready with your concerns and questions. It is a good idea to note these down in advance. Clear communication from both sides is essential to build a partnership. Today, oncologists are no longer the only source of information about cancer. The internet, for one, is full of valuable information and, if carefully studied, will answer most of your preliminary concerns and questions. Cancer support groups have also mushroomed in all major cities. They are well-trained to cope with most of our needs.

As far as possible, always visit your oncologist with a family member or friend. Two heads are better than one in coping with health questions that you might find complex. And as time progresses, as the partnership grows, you yourself may

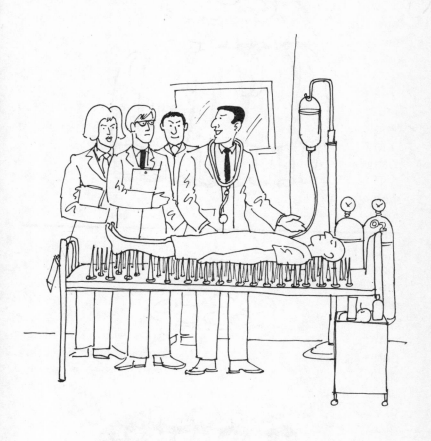

"And this is the ward where we mix alternative medicine with chemotherapy."

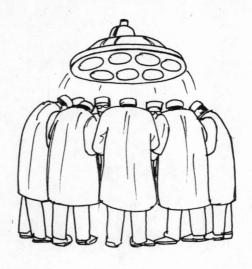

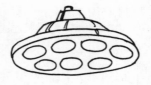

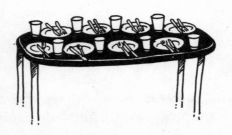

be able to treat minor setbacks in the treatment without bothering your oncologist. Cancer patients are extremely vulnerable and tend to become more and more dependent on their oncologists. But never forget who is in command. Whose health and life is at stake. Always be in control and learn to help yourself as much as possible. A second opinion can be of great help but can also show lack of trust and faith in the selected team of medical advisers. Never get intimidated by a doctor. Communication is of utmost importance. Tell the oncologist all he would want to know. Tell him more than what you think he would want to know. Unless you communicate, he will never know what your health status is. Participate in your treatment. Take the lead. It's up to you to build the partnership.

Frequent blood tests were necessary after each chemotherapy cycle. We decided to use a laboratory closer to home. Most often I was able to drive down myself but there were times when I felt weak and exhausted and nurses had to come home for a blood sample. Once the blood sample had been given, a long wait began. At times, the five to six hours required for the reports to be ready seemed like five to six years. I used to get nervous and irritated. If the blood was not up to the mark, a series of injections were necessary. Or even hospitalization. Or blood transfusion. Blood tests were repeated just before it was time for the next chemotherapy cycle to begin. If the parameters were not up to the mark, the chemotherapy was postponed. The long treatment can become even longer in this manner.

Chemotherapy started on June 10, 2000. After that day, I took total control. The time that had elapsed had given me the wisdom to learn from my own mistakes, from the mistakes of other patients, and also from mistakes of the medical profession. With cancer, there is no time to be wasted. The treatment must begin the moment the diagnosis is complete. It's advisable to put the rest of your life on hold as you focus on making important treatment decisions. On choosing not just the treatment but also the right doctors. This is the difficult period. You, your family and your friends, may still be recovering from the shock of the diagnosis. Knowledge levels may be poor. Talking to other cancer patients and learning from their experiences is not always that easy. In any case, each patient is different. Each cancer is unique.

As decisions on the treatment get finalized, a greater sense of urgency comes in. You seem to be in greater control, ready to lead your troops from the front. The initial fright of the diagnosis slowly starts to disappear. You feel more confident in your efforts to win the war. There is no way of knowing that the course of treatment you select is the best. There is no way of knowing for instance, if the combination of chemotherapy and ayurvedic medicines, supported by reiki healing, is the best form of medication for all cancer patients. What is most critical is how soon you are able to move into a treatment mode and build on your acceptance levels so as to wholeheartedly participate in that treatment. Once having decided on the course of treatment, try not to look back. Not unless there is a real reason to do so.

Patience is critical. You can never tell when some part of your treatment will get postponed. And even when the first stage of the treatment is over, it can be extended further, depending on the response. I still remember the agonizing wait after my chest x-ray was taken at the end of the second chemotherapy cycle. The results of the x-ray would determine my response to the chemotherapy. I paced up and down like a lunatic. At one stage my oncologist suggested I be given a mild sedative. It was Amrita, as always, who calmed my nerves.

Synergy between all medical advisers is of course ideal, but if for some reason there is disagreement, as happened in my case, between my oncologist and my ayurvedic adviser, it is the patient who should make the final decision. The body undergoing treatment responds in many different and peculiar ways. And most of the time provides the patient with answers that medical advisers may not always be in agreement with. In my case, my oncologist was against my continuing with ayurvedic treatment. Her reasoning was that she did not know what I was being given and it could therefore interfere with the chemotherapy drug and complicate matters. She was right in her way of thinking. However, when I took second and third opinions from other experts and even cancer patients, I came to the conclusion that I should continue with the ayurvedic treatment as long as my body could cope with it. Of course, I did not breathe a word to my oncologist. I came to the conclusion that I was as responsible for my eventual well-being as she was. My success would also be her success.

Be creative in your approach to your treatment. Think of ways and means to stay ahead of your cancer. Live life to the fullest, but that does not mean that you strain yourself. And don't worry about how your grandparents found their solutions. It's your body. It's your mind. It's your cancer. It's your battle. Only you have the answers to how you can win.

*Only you and I
can help the sun rise each coming morning.
If we don't,
it might drench itself out in sorrow.*

Joan Baez

BATTLE PLAN 3
THINKING POSITIVE

I was in the ICU after surgery, heavily drugged. There was excruciating pain in the left side of my chest. I could hear people talking in hushed voices. For the life of me I couldn't make out what they were saying. I opened my eyes and the world was a blur. Someone was trying to hold my hand. The pain was unbearable. I drifted back to sleep and then woke up again. Both the surgeon, Dr. Chaturvedi and Amrita were leaning over me, trying to say something. From her face I could make out that all was not right.

I began to feel cheated. I felt anger. I felt deep remorse. All sorts of equipment were still attached to me to help me with my breathing. I felt trapped. I couldn't speak. I couldn't ask questions. It was a nightmare. Amrita stayed by my bed the entire night, simply stroking my head, hushing me up gently every time I made an effort to speak. Though she said nothing, the expression on her face told me everything. The cancer had spread. None of this had emerged in the innumerable tests that were done prior to the surgery. And of course, the huge 35 cm scar would remain, like a deep gash dividing my body into two, an eternal reminder of the fallibility of medical treatment. My mind rebelled. I was furious.

The next day, I was informed that I would have to undergo

chemotherapy. The very sound of that word sent shivers down my spine. Images of my mother coping with her chemotherapy kept haunting me. For her, and for all of us who supported her those days, it was an unending nightmare. Of pain. Of discomfort. Of an unimaginable living hell. Amrita and my friends tried to console me by saying that considerable progress had been made by medical science since then. All that helped to calm my nerves, but fear and anger continued to stalk me. Did I have it in me to cope with the long and arduous journey that lay ahead. I had no other option. I had to muster up all my mental and physical resources to be able to cope. With grace. And with dignity.

It was then that I made the decision to be an active participant in my treatment. Participate in as creative a manner as was possible. I knew the cancer cells had a haphazard existence. I decided to remain positive at all stages and use all my mental and physical energies to ensure that I would remain in control. The unnecessary surgery, and the thought of the permanent scar that I would have to live with, had somewhat weakened my resolve to fight back. This was a luxury that I just could not afford. Even in their haphazard behaviour, the cancer cells still controlled my life. There was a definite method in their madness. Where did they get their strength? How were they able to sustain their onslaught? Especially when they existed and survived in a manner that defied the laws of nature. Nature has a definite pattern, and this pattern repeats itself without any variation through the years, for centuries. A set of laws that govern every aspect of the complex universe. Yet cancer cells, without adhering to any rules, survive and proliferate, creating havoc. They controlled the remaining years of my life. They made their own laws. So, how could anyone get the better of such abnormal behavior? How could I wrest control again?

The conclusion I arrived at was that the only way to win was to totally confuse the cancer cells by being creative in my attack. Being defensive was a sure sign of weakness. Beating them at their own game by being as haphazard as them was just not the answer. They were the masters of such behaviour. I had to attack them in a manner that was totally alien to them. A number of patients that I had come across at the hospital had allowed themselves to be overtaken by their cancer. The disease had not only created havoc in their physical selves but had also managed to attack and break down their mental and emotional well-being. They appeared as if all their inner strength had been sapped and were just about able to complete the motions of daily living. Cancer had eaten into their mind-body continuum and their willingness to fight back just did not exist. This was all too apparent in their reactions and responses. The way they slowly and aimlessly trudged along the hospital corridors. As if a pall of gloom hung over their heads. They were just not able to cope with the rigours of the war. They were heavily battle-scarred and totally disoriented. Those accompanying them had fallen into the same syndrome.

I decided to sustain the war in an organized manner. Confuse the malignant cells with my inner strength. Beat them by being least affected by their presence. I had heard stories about how the treatment for cancer was far worse than cancer itself. It was clear that all mental and physical reserves would be required in order to stay ahead at all times. I had to be positive. I had to think positive. No matter when the worst side effects of chemotherapy surfaced and in what form to bring down my defenses. Shatter my reinforcements.

Those were the war games I played, the tactics that I

employed, as the first drops of Taxotere flowed into my system through the intravenous drip. And the Cisplatin the next day. And during the subsequent cycles that followed. My immunity level dropped to an alarmingly low level. My nausea became more and more uncontrollable. My appetite and food intake decreased and there were days when I couldn't keep down even a sip of water. I continued to lose weight. As the chemotherapy treatment progressed, friends and family around me started to despair. But my resolve remained. Some of my worst moments I overcame by thinking about how cancer had benefited me. I relived the good and joyous moments in my life. I stayed positive. Filled my mind with strong creative thoughts and desires that could bring me joy. It wasn't easy. At times, almost impossible. As the days went by I discovered an unimaginable reservoir of energy that existed somewhere deep inside. Something that I thought I never had in me. Something that just came together.

It was during this period that I made it clear to all around me that I was not willing to cope with any negativity in my surroundings. As soon as Amrita realized that even the slightest degree of negativity made me somewhat falter in my resolve, even minor matters that might have adversely effected my mental state were not brought to my notice. When our car met with an accident and was badly damaged I was told about it much later when all the repairs were over. As also the fire in the kitchen. The breakup of the marriage of one of my best friends. The bills that had to be paid. I was living in an ivory tower filled with only positive energies. Positive thoughts. This wasn't easy on Amrita. On my children. On my relatives and friends. At times everything around seemed so unreal. But I was grateful for all the support and encouragement that I received. Some people called me selfish. Others said I was running away from reality. But I too was carrying a heavy burden. All my energies were focused at the task at hand. And the task was gigantic. At times it appeared insurmountable. I was convinced that living with a positive attitude was the only way that I could succeed. Change my karma. Alter my mother's karma. So that the generations that followed did not have to go through what I was going through.

The truth is that cancer, at most times, is self-inflicted. Long periods of stress are considered a major cause. Diet is another. So are smoking and consumption of other tobacco products. Genetic disorders may also lead to cancer. Industrialization, exposure to radiation and pollution are known to cause cancer. But all this happens only when the human immune system breaks down. When the mind and body are no longer in sync. And to overcome cancer, the mind and body must fight in unison. A holistic approach is essential. Every mind has its own unique body. Every body also has a unique mind. The body we can see, feel and touch. The mind is something we only sense. But deep down, in our subconscious, we can relate to them together as one single entity. When the body is afflicted, the mind alone can never undo the damage. Together they must fight back to win control. And it is this leap into the subconscious that is crucial. There are greater chances of success if all our forces are united. The complex laws of duality govern nature. One without the other and all is lost. In the war against cancer, the mind-body continuum must obey the principle of duality, especially since cancer cells proliferate and survive in a haphazard manner. But how can the cancer patient bring together the mind-body connection? Meditation helps. So does introspection. And most of all, being positive even during the worst moments of the treatment.

I decided to delve deeper into my subconscious. Hours of chanting. *Nam-myoho-renge-kyo*. The basic practice of the Buddhism of Nichiren Daishonin. Supported by the daily practice of morning and evening *gongyo*, the recitation of the two key chapters of the Lotus Sutra. By studying the Buddhist way of life, a state in which all desires are completely fulfilled and developed. This created the maximum value and good fortune for myself and for the others who supported me, accompanied by an unshakable happiness and confidence, regardless of the existing problems. It is in tackling a powerful enemy that one's real strength is fully   realized. Put simply, the teachings of Buddhism showed me how the desire to overcome suffering was one of the greatest incentives for overall progress. The chanting of *nam-myoho-renge-kyo* helped in changing my karma. *Myoho-renge-kyo* literally means 'mystic law of the Lotus Sutra' and *nam* is a verbal contraction of the Sanskrit word *nama* or *namas*, meaning devotion. Thus *nam-myoho-renge-kyo* can be said to mean 'I devote my life to the mystic law of the Lotus Sutra'.

And meditation. *Shrava asana* from among the yoga *asanas*. Reiki healing. And *yoga nidra*. Devotional music. Hours would pass by in such a manner every night. And many a time, I fell into a deep sleep. Many a time, Amrita would switch off the music that I had got so used to listening to until the early hours of the morning. Often I felt that all my mental and physical energies were totally drained. Often I felt that I just did not have the strength to live to fight another day. Often I felt myself being reduced to a state of non-being. But I persisted. Till a divine state of peace engulfed me. Till the room was full of only positive energy. Till I had journeyed deep into my subconscious. Till the mind and body came together to fight the enemy. Till I could reason with the cancer cells. Make peace with them, unmindful of their haphazard behaviour. A prewar negotiation and dialogue as it were. At times I succeeded. At other times I know I failed. Yet my persistence must have worked more often than not. At times there was unbearable pain. At other times I felt nothing. And with the pain, I could feel the improvement in my lungs. I had to motivate my lungs, the battleground, to throw out the infiltrators that were so deeply entrenched. Each day, I was participating in my own healing. It was something as strong and powerful as my medication. As the chemotherapy drugs that were being administered every three weeks. It was a cure that sprang from a source that was deep inside me. The same source that had brought my mind and body together. I was convinced that my cancer was self-inflicted. And that only I possessed the energy, the strength and the holistic approach to take charge and be rid of it. Each day and each night I persisted. Hoping that I would eventually be a part of the ten percent group of patients who successfully responded to chemotherapy for lung cancer.

Most cancer patients that I spoke to did not realize the importance of this holistic approach. The togetherness of the mind and body. The hazardous journey into the subconscious. Hazardous since it requires vast amounts of positive energy. Positive thinking. An important aspect of any treatment and cure. Even minor ones for that matter. We do not focus on our inner being, our mind-body continuum, and use its true potential. Our hidden strengths that need to be activated. In most cases, we are quick to blame the outside world for the state we are in. It is easy for most of us to take credit for good fortune, but only a few are willing to accept complete blame for any ills. As long as the going is good, all is well and the mind-body continuum continues to flourish. The moment even a small tragedy strikes, even the strongest amongst us gets shattered. It is during these moments that our inner strength needs to come into play. Unfortunately, we are quick to seek external help and guidance. Very rarely do we use the mind-body continuum to help resolve the crisis that we are faced with.

We have all heard and read about miracle cures. In books. In real life. Even with serious cancer patients. And in other conditions of poor health. Miracle cures have been known for centuries. Yet if we are to believe in the cause and effect theory, every miracle cure has to have a cause. And this cause, more often than not, begins from within. And the marshalling of all the forces that reside within us. Miracle cures are often the end result of the mind and body coming together. Of our own inner strength. A positive attitude that must begin from the day of the diagnosis. The utilization of our own energies to participate in our own health program.

When we change our inner thoughts, feelings and attitudes, our outer experiences automatically change. There is a definite relationship between what goes on inside us and what happens in our external world. This understanding is the beginning of bringing the mind and body to work together to overcome anything that may have unsettled our basic equilibrium. Cancer, or even any minor ailment for that matter, upsets the balance of the mind-body continuum. Nothing can happen on the outside till it first surfaces on the inside. The coming together and the perfect balance of the mind-body continuum relaxes the mind, rebuilds the body. When we control our mind and body, we control our entire world. Cancer can be the result of destructive mental and emotional attitudes. In the early stages, cancer shows up as weakness and lack of immunity of some kind. Allowed to continue undetected and uncontrolled in most cases, the negative forces gradually wear down and destroy the equilibrium of the mind-body continuum. However, if we cooperate with the life force that exists within each one of us, the alignment of the mind-body takes control and the destructive forces get negated, thereby allowing the body to rebuild itself. According to an ancient Chinese proverb 'he who conquers a city is great, he who conquers himself is mighty'.

The importance of the togetherness of the mind and body in the war against cancer should never be underestimated. After hours and days of trying to relax the mind and body, I found my own way of regaining my equilibrium. By taking the mind off everything that had been of any major consequence in my life before I was stricken by the disease. Relaxation and deep breathing helped. So did adequate rest and sleep backed by proper scheduling of all activities. Some days, I spent hours communicating with nature. Staring at the birds. Healing myself through their joy, their chirping and the simplicity in their behaviour. Watching flowers bloom. Total emptiness of the mind. Complete relaxation of the body. Readjustment of the mind and body. Coming together. Fighting together. The holistic approach. I don't remember exactly when everything started changing. The mind and body in total sync. All I can recall is that there was a time when I felt that my cancer had begun to regress. That a few of the many battles had been won. Of course there were many, many more miles to go.

The unity of the mind and body is all encompassing. And if for some reason there is great resentment inside you, especially as a result of your cancer, the sooner you can overcome it the better it will be for your treatment and recovery.

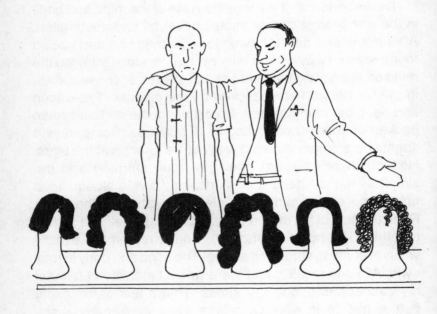

"Look at it this way, now you can change your hairstyle every day of the week."

A cancer patient knows that it is not easy to be positive and remain positive all along, especially during the side effects of the treatment. After the initial shock of the diagnosis, it takes a great deal of effort to be positive. At these early stages, you may not be able to forgive yourself for what has happened. You may want to vent your anger, your resentment, on those around you. On your friends and   family. On all those who would support you in the long and arduous days of the treatment. You may feel victimized. Not just by them. By the treatment. By your health. And most of all by yourself. Soon, a stage may be reached where the resentment and anger is not just a part of you, but also creeps into the people around you. Always remember that resentment causes stress. And stress causes cancer cells to flourish.

You cannot afford such self-indulgence. There is no time for such 'luxuries'. Remember, there are those who will recover and be cured, and unfortunately, there are also those who will succumb to the cancer, even though the diagnosis and the treatment may be similar. The former always consider the present as just an aberration that will pass and look forward to many years of healthy living post the treatment. They spend most of their time pondering over all the good things that cancer has led to. How cancer has benefited them. And the millions of things they would achieve once their treatment is completed. As cancer patients, we all have our own stories to tell. How cancer has changed our life. Dwell on the bright side. It goes a long way towards total cure. It changes the way you look at yourself. At your cancer. It gives you courage and energy to do things that you have never done before. To do the same things, but to do them differently. And in so doing, it builds on your positive attitudes. Sustains them over longer periods. And gives you the will to outlive your cancer. At most times, your mind is activated and involved with things that are closely connected with your cancer. There are other things in life which are equally important.

You should not even for a moment allow the cancer to overtake you. Fight hard to postpone any bout of negativity that attempts to enter the environment. Anything that can affect you adversely. Remind yourself of the thousands of reasons why you must continue to live. And fight. This realization must come from within.

We are each of us angels with only one wing;
and we can only fly by embracing one another.

Luciano de Crescenzo

BATTLE PLAN 4

HARNESSING THE SUPPORT OF FAMILY AND FRIENDS

News of my cancer spreads like wildfire, amongst family and friends. As soon as I returned from Mumbai, I had a stream of visitors, some that I had not set my eyes on since childhood. All meaning well. All with some advice to offer. Each had his or her story to tell. Their own brush with cancer. A friend who had recovered. A relative who was under treatment. They wanted to know what I was going through. How I would cope. What my thoughts were. And soon enough, though visitors were always welcome, I began to get tired. Exhausted with the never-ending stories. Tired of making polite conversation when actually I wanted to hide from everyone. From the entire world around me. I felt I had been disfigured. I felt it would take a long time for me to contribute significantly to society. Seeing them, meeting them, I started feeling low. How could they continue with their lives as if nothing had happened? For me, life would never be the same again.

Those who came showered me with love, care and concern. At times I thought it was more, much more, than what I deserved. They expressed solidarity during this critical stage of my life. At times friends had to be turned away because I was exhausted. At times, the chemotherapy drugs reduced my immunity to alarmingly low levels and barrier nursing was essential. Without any fuss or hurt those people returned later to express concern, to ask what I was going through. All this helped. All this made my resolve to win my war against cancer stronger. I could not let them down. I had to live up to their expectations. Their words of solace. Their words of advice.

I do realize that everyone is not so fortunate. There are cancer patients who fight their war single-handedly or with minimal support from friends and family. I had met quite a few such patients during my numerous trips to the hospital. I introduced them to cancer support groups that I had been in touch with. Lent them books they could read about their disease. Downloaded information from various websites.

Such conversations at the hospital affected me in their own way. They reminded me of those among my friends and family who never came. Initially I was glad they didn't add to the unending stream of visitors. Later I concluded that they just did not care. As each day passed, and the possibility of their visit receded further, a sense of resignation overtook me. But somewhere deep down it hurt. Why had they forsaken me at a time when I most needed their support? I had to remind myself that all of us have our own lives to lead. Have our own share of problems. Obviously what was of great importance to me was not of any great significance to them. Had I wronged them in any manner in the past? Maybe I *did* matter but they were preoccupied with matters of greater importance in their lives. After some time they just did not matter. As far as I was concerned, nothing else mattered but my war against cancer. And more and more as time went by, the anger against them that was simmering inside subsided.

My father too showed no concern. We lived in the same city but he didn't even telephone to find out how I was progressing. Initially I told myself he was old and frail. He was losing his memory. As the days turned into weeks and the weeks into months, there was still no communication from my father. It hurt deeply. Had he abandoned me? Had the cancer anything to do with it? Had he treated my mother in a similar manner when she was fighting her cancer? Halfway through my treatment I decided to meet him. Confront him with how I felt. I was meeting him after more than five months. He had changed. He looked older and more frail than before. He had no answers. Since our finances were dwindling, I asked him for some help, a temporary loan, which he refused.

All this caused tremendous pain and grief. It resulted in unnecessary stress. I thought a lot about the people, the friends and relatives, who had showed total lack of concern. I remembered the amount of time and effort Amrita and I had devoted to them when they were in trouble. People who just did not find the time during my hour of need. Had I misunderstood them? Had Amrita and I over-stepped and done more for them than what was necessary? Had we been wrong in assuming that they cared as much for us as we did for them? Yes it really hurt. It aroused a sense of deep resentment against them. And against my own self. And when the resentment started to change towards negativity, that is when I realized that such people did not and should not matter to me at all.

I could not afford any negativity in my environment. I had to at all times be positive in mind, body and soul. I decided that I would have very little to do with them in the future. And no amount of explanation or reasons for their lack of concern would ever suffice to overcome the pain and hurt they had caused. The absence of support from a few quarters can cause greater pain and stress than the joy and comfort you feel from an unending stream of visitors showering you with love, care and concern.

People are different. People change. They react differently when a friend or a relative has a serious health problem. Some are warm and show endless care and concern. Others find it difficult to accept, but manage to build up just about sufficient strength and courage to show concern. And then there are those who just shy away from any form of adversity. For the patient, this is extremely difficult to accept. On most days, my life began and ended only with my health status. Some found this to be extremely selfish, but only I knew how much strength was needed to think beyond my own health condition. Especially beyond cancer.

What you communicate is what others will communicate with you. When you project positive vibrations all around, everyone is positive. And when you succumb to the agonies and the trials and tribulations of the treatment, your friends will also convey misery and agony. The best thing for you and for them is to spread good cheer all around you. And from the good cheer you receive, you derive more joy and happiness. The strength that you need to keep your mind and body together, so as to win the war that you set out to win. You, the cancer patient, are in command of how others around you react to your joys and pain, to your treatment, to your winning the war. And remember always that winning a war is a collective effort. No one has won a war single-handedly. Short skirmishes, possibly. But a full-fledged war, never. Eventually it is the collective strength of everyone involved, of every single participant, that gets you to win that war.

The most difficult aspect of this war is to be able to think beyond yourself and your own selfish needs and of being wanted by everyone all the time. I could manage it only for a few short moments. And in those moments, the grief that my cancer was causing all around would overcome my concern for my own self. There were times I wanted to be alone with myself, my thoughts. Sometimes I bolted the bedroom door from inside. I had to be alone. I just could not let people around me see me weaken. I didn't want to cast a pall of gloom all around. So all alone, all by myself, I lay in bed. Thinking of the grief, the agony, my cancer was causing. These moments came and these moments passed. And never was I able to share them with anyone. I didn't know if anyone would understand. Whether I understood anyone either. Some, who at times thought I was being selfish. If only they knew how my heart wanted to reach out to them. If only they could see how grieved I was with the whole situation.

It's not just you, the patient, who gets deeply affected. The lives of all the members of the family change. There are those who will go out of their way to show care and concern. And some who will willingly sacrifice their own lives, their valuable time, to help out. And some who may not feel the same way. And stay aloof. All this should not be cause for worry. Accept it as a part of life. Do not question, in any manner, the ways of the world. Cancer is a destructive disease. It starts with destroying the internal cells of the afflicted. Continues the internal destruction, unnoticed and without any external symptoms. At some stage or other, the cancer is diagnosed. A routine examination. Or a special cancer checkup. Then it begins to affect the patient's life. And the lives of all those who are close. The immediate family members. The spouse.

The children. The relatives. Close friends. Not just through the discomfort of accompanying the patient in the many hospital trips that are necessary and the changes that are to be made in their own schedules. Or by the mental torture arising from the fact that someone extremely close to them might be dying. Cancer works in its own haphazard manner. It does not play by any of the rules that we are familiar with. When it will strike, where and how, no one can predict. But when it strikes, it devastates the patient. And then in its own devious ways, those who are close. As I was beginning to discover.

I still remember so clearly how Amrita used to raise and lower my hospital bed. During the many days that I had to stay in hospital. Before and after my surgery. My chemotherapy. All that and more were beginning to affect her back. And one day, she could not bear the excruciating pain any more. All that while she had suffered in silence. Ignoring something that had needed immediate attention. Sacrificing her pain for the sake of mine. One day she had to be rushed to hospital where her pain was diagnosed as the beginnings of a slipped disc. She spent three days undergoing tests. Here was my chance to look after her. The way she had laboured over me all those days. But it was just not possible. I was too weak and my immunity levels so low that I was told not to even think of going anywhere near a hospital. When Amrita returned home she was advised complete bed rest for three weeks. We coped with the situation to the best of our ability. The room was reorganized. Instead of one patient, there were two patients in the house now. A nurse used to come every day to assist her in the mornings. Her sister, Shiela, flew in from the Gulf to look after us.

Shiela took over from Amrita. She accompanied me on

my hospital trips. When I had to undergo minor surgery at the time the chemo-port was installed. During my chemotherapy cycles. She brought good cheer into our devastated lives. She joked. She laughed. She played on our piano. She sang. She looked into my diet. Brought fresh dates from her garden in Muscat. I will never forget the many varieties of the most delicious soups that she prepared for me. Sip by sip I drank, a few sips every hour. Since nothing else was being retained by my body as a result of the nausea.

Even my daughters' lives were badly affected. The younger one, Kaveri, had just graduated. She had planned to go abroad for further studies. My cancer changed all that. Instead she decided to get a job. Postponing her plans to study further until I recovered. Her life was reduced to working and looking after me. Most of the nights that I spent in hospital, she was there with me. I felt sorry for her. A young girl. Full of life and energy. Spending evening after evening taking care of her cancer-ridden father. And when her friends came to see her, instead of going out with them, she stayed at home. Even my elder daughter, Malika, had to cope with devastation in her personal life, brought on by her father's illness and all that it entailed for the family.

I tried to share their grief. It wasn't easy with what I was going through myself. It is extremely important that all lines of communications be open at all times. The best way for the cancer patient to achieve this is to act normal and natural. This is easier said than done. You are the one fighting for your life, so how can you behave normally? How can you behave in the same manner as you did before? You can't just overlook the presence of cancer cells in your body. But if you think rationally, why should the presence of some malignant cells change everyone's life, torment a whole family? Have such a drastic influence on everyone? In order to come to terms with cancer, the first thing is to accept its presence. This is a period that could be charged with emotion and many of the feelings may not seem appropriate or acceptable. At times there may be anger. Or wanting to run far away from it all. It is imperative that no judgment is passed on these feelings which may fluctuate from one end of the spectrum to the other. Moods can swing in a matter of a few minutes. All that needs to be done is to gracefully accept what is happening in your environment and not pass judgement. The cancer should never be given too much importance. And there are no right or wrong kind of feelings. None that are mature or immature. They are all just feelings.

As a cancer patient, you can go through great swings of mood. You can experience fear, anger, self-pity, remorse, and joy ... all in a matter of minutes. The emotional ups and downs can be frightening. You must ensure that the people around learn to cope with such variable moods. Provide the reassurance that is required even at times of great adversity. There is a greater tendency for families and friends to be most loving, supportive and caring when you are weak and helpless. And need all the looking after that is required. As soon as you feel a bit better, you are left to your own devices. It is imperative that you act in as independent a manner as is physically possible when you are in a weak and vulnerable condition. If all the love and caring is showered on you when you are weak, your self-healing and your own initiatives in improving your health weaken. The disease should never be glorified, should not be rewarded with added help and support. Your own initiatives to improve your health should be supported. You should be encouraged to be as self-sufficient as possible. This is what builds your reserves of positive

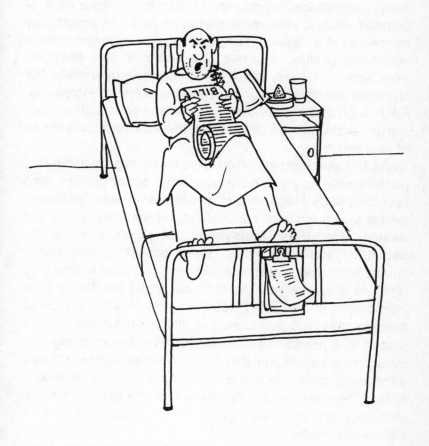

"Now I know why they wear masks in hospitals."

energy. So always try and cope with adversity to the best of your own ability. It is easy to succumb to the support of people around you in moments of weakness. Thereby, you virtually deny yourself the opportunity of learning to take care of yourself. Always remember that such kind of support only reinforces the illness. The best way to emerge from a vulnerable position is to use your energies, your strength, from within. This will zap a lot of your energy initially, but ultimately you will find your own reserves of energy increasing. Each such attempt should be construed as a sign of your own inner strength and a bold step towards the improvement of your health.

As and when you are physically able to do so, you need to participate in your normal range of activities and responsibilities. Helplessness, or worse still, an unnecessary desire for continuous handholding, is something that will destroy your inner resolve and strength. Even when bedridden, you are in a much better position to discuss the course your treatment should take. And you must make every effort to preserve your normal role within the family unit. Participate in all family activities. Ward off feelings of helplessness and abandonment. It's a terrible thing to be placed in a position of dependency. Apart from being life-threatening, cancer can also destroy your self-esteem. Every effort must be made not to compound your helplessness further. Normal living patterns within the family unit are extremely important not just for the long term, but also for day-to-day coping.

Yes, under treatment, life can get totally disrupted. If this is allowed to happen for a long period of time, it becomes even more difficult to resume normal family functioning during the subsequent periods of remission or cure. People around you will always have the desire to 'do something' and it is this very desire that you must curtail. Cancer is easier to live with and accept if everyone is as constructive as possible. To make each day count for what they have put into it together.

On such a full sea are we now afloat
And we must take the current when it serves
Or lose our ventures.

Shakespeare in *Julius Ceasar*

BATTLE PLAN 5
SETTING GOALS

One night I just couldn't sleep. A deep resentment was setting in since the feeling that the doctors had experimented with my body was getting stronger day by day. How could different doctors have such different interpretations of the same set of data? The doctors in Mumbai had ruled out surgery at the eleventh hour. Two sets of doctors in Delhi had independently suggested that surgery was the better option. As I lay in bed, with some amount of discomfort in the right side of my chest, my mind wandered. It dwelt on various incidents in my life that had been of great significance. My first cricket bat which was gifted to me when I only eight years old. And how I thought at that time that I would be the next Bradman of the game. My first job and how excited I was when I received the appointment letter. My marriage and the birth of our first daughter. Our first holiday as a family outside the shores of India and the excitement on the faces of our children as we set foot on another land far away from home. But now lay what ahead? This was the question that kept coming back to me over and over again. There was so much that I still wanted to do. There was so much that I still wanted to see. I wanted to travel in outer space and experience weightlessness. I wanted to trek further and further in the Himalayas so that I could be one with nature. I wanted to work in an office again, something that my cancer had denied me. So many things whizzed past my mind. Things I had not accomplished but had always wanted to. Some of them were simple things. Some were dreams that I knew would never be fulfilled. Some I just had to accomplish. That night I decided that I wouldn't let cancer destroy my capacity to dream. That night I decided that at the start of each day I would set myself a goal, an objective, for that day. And ensure that more often than not it was achieved. I began with daily objectives, and soon there were objectives for the week, the month, the year. And also for the many years of life that I had promised myself.

In the months that followed I made frequent visits to the hospital. There were long sessions of chemotherapy. Waiting for my turn to come. My name to be announced. Like a lamb being taken to the slaughterhouse. Talking to other cancer patients who were in a similar condition as I was. I concentrated on the ones who were responding well to the treatment. Winning their daily battles against cancer. I tried to find out what set them apart from those who had not been so successful. They all had strong reasons to live. They could elaborate their reasons in great detail. They too, like me, felt that this strong urge to be alive was the single most important explanation for their positive response to the treatment.

Their reasons for wanting to be alive were as simple or as meaningful as mine. From participating in the growing up of their grandchild to enjoying the unknown and hoping for additional benefits in the new millennium. From ensuring that their new house was fully constructed to meeting a son who was returning from America later in the year. Some even talked about the day their dog would give birth to her pups. The flowers that would bloom in their garden in the forthcoming spring. The graduation day ceremony of their daughter. All had a special meaning. Each one was of great significance for the patient. And each objective, each goal led to another. Allowing them to stay ahead. And then setting themselves a new set of goals. Their dreams giving them just that little extra to win the war. That little bit of extra will power that was so essential to tilt the balance in their favour. Giving them that added inner strength. And the joy of having lived another day.

What was so simple and taken for granted before their diagnosis meant so much now. A greater effort was required in living each day, and each passing day had so much meaning for them. Something that was unique to each individual and held no meaning for any other. Most people take life for granted. On a daily basis, people don't even bother to speculate about what lies ahead. Tomorrow. Or the next week. Or a year from now. Maybe five years ahead. Yet the same people, when they, or any of their loved ones, are faced with a life-threatening disease like cancer, find themselves contemplating the times ahead. When cancer strikes, it changes the course of so many lives. Goals in life change. Cancer patients are no longer in any position to take their lives for granted. Time is not in their hands any more. Planning for five years ahead, which they could do so easily earlier, no longer has the same relevance.

Setting daily goals and objectives within the overall longer-term plan helps. Especially when the treatment for control and cure is a major part of daily life. Goals and objectives need to be redefined. The will to live is stronger when there is something to look forward to and live for. A greater effort has to be made to achieve things that you want from life. Setting goals and attempting to achieve those goals helps in channelizing your energies. It gives a sharper focus to all your activities. Accepting your cancer and coping with its treatment becomes that much easier. You, the patient, are in charge of your own life. And this raises your self-esteem. You feel proud at having achieved what you set out to. In little ways it all adds up. Making you more confident. Preparing your mental, physical and emotional faculties to work together for the daily assaults. Bringing the mind and body together. Making each passing day a joyous one. Building your reserves to achieve your ultimate goal. You rediscover the joys of accomplishment. Of achieving simple objectives which in turn can lead to harnessing the more difficult ones.

A word of caution. There may be times when your objectives are not achieved. And this could lead you to a state of depression. You could feel like a non-achiever. The fear of failure should strengthen your resolve further. Life was never meant to be easy, and now more so as a cancer patient. This is the time to remember that striving to meet your goals is as important as actually achieving them. After all, your goals and objectives are just another method of channelizing your inner strength and energy. Of ensuring that you are not led astray from a single-minded resolve. And this is of greater significance than if a few of your daily goals are left unfulfilled. Your goals get altered as your priorities change. New ones will constantly get added, others dropped. Only you understand your needs and requirements for the day. If some of your objectives are not being fulfilled, either you are striving too high or not enough effort is being made on your part. While it is important for your self-esteem that your objectives are met, it is equally important that you continue to work towards achieving your goals. The results of your daily efforts may bring a great amount of satisfaction.

And unless you are focused, your energies will get dissipated.

As a cancer patient, your life changes forever. Not just your life but also the lives of all who are close to you. You need clarity on what is important and you need to focus on it. The zest for living and a sense of joy, creativity and spontaneity acquire greater meaning than ever before. Brooding and complaining will only draw you further into the 'Why *me*?' syndrome. The more positive and hopeful you are, the less energy it takes to produce better results in improving your health. All you have to do is to explore new ways of spending your day. Continue your efforts to meet a new set of objectives that will add excitement to your life. This sheer force of commitment will contribute in a big way to producing results. Every little thought or action adds up.

Living through one difficult day can seem much longer than even six months of life without cancer. An hour of the first chemotherapy session can be the longest span of time possible. But then each moment must pass. And soon each chemotherapy session becomes a routine. Like the way a man has to shave every morning. Why was it that the first session of chemotherapy seemed much longer to me than the sixty minutes it took for the drug to flow? Apart from the fear and anxiety, I didn't have my goals clearly defined. The same experience however, was never repeated. In the subsequent sessions, I was prepared. There was less fear and anxiety. And above all, a well-defined objective that helped the mind-body continuum to accept the drugs faster. And better. Even before the drugs began to flow, efforts towards achieving the established objectives had already been initiated. I was in full control, having gained knowledge and wisdom from the previous experience. The mind-body continuum too was more receptive, more accommodating of the drugs.

Working towards achieving long-term goals can at times be frustrating. The more long-term they are, the greater the effort required. As time passes by, you could experience a sense of failure. In the long waiting period, you could get side-tracked. As a cancer patient, your long-term goal is to be cured and remain disease-free for the remaining years of your life. Cancer is the centre-stage of your life. Under normal circumstances, cancer does not usually enter your scheme of things. For the first 50 years of my life, cancer was never a major issue. However, in the last few months, any small news item about cancer, any experience of even a distant friend or relative … everything and anything related to the disease attracted my attention immediately. My objectives had changed. Yes, my prime purpose was to be cancer-free as soon as possible and for as long as possible. But I realized that this would take its own time. And in this period, I had to set myself other objectives to keep my spirits high. Ensure that my morale did not sag. And even when it did, which I knew it would, and also had at times as a result of the side effects of the treatment, I had to have my own therapy ready to bring it back on track.

I remember the time just about a few weeks ago, when my immunity levels were so low as a result of the side effects of the chemotherapy drugs that I had to be isolated and kept under observation. In a 100% sterile environment, with no visitors. As I lay in bed, as masked doctors and nurses rushed in and out of the room, as more and more antibiotics flowed into my system so as to prevent infection, my priorities for the moment changed. Cancer and its treatment took a back seat. For those three days I fought hard and used all my energy to keep infection at bay. My objectives had shifted.

This three-day stay at the hospital confirmed my worst fears about the treatment. Right from the beginning my oncologist had advised me to try and avoid crowded places. Busy shopping centres. Cinema halls. Airports and railway stations. For fear of catching infection. As a result of the side effects of the chemotherapy drugs, immunity levels can fall to alarmingly low levels. This makes you highly susceptible to all sorts of infection. With my bald head and protective mask that covered most of my face, I must have looked a sight. All this discouraged me to leave my room, my home, very often. I lost the desire to venture into the world outside my doorstep. My exercises were reduced to walking inside the house. Or deep breathing during my meditation and chanting hours. Sometimes I was not allowed to meet even the small groups of people, my friends, who came to visit me. I felt the loneliness of the long distance runner. Alone and scared of what lay ahead. What helped me at each of those times was the renewal of goals and objectives. And striving hard to achieve them.

The situation changed somewhat when I landed myself a short three-month consultancy assignment. The costs of the treatment had drained our finances. We were sinking deeper and deeper in debt. It was sheer stroke of luck when I received a call from a friend. The organization that he was working with required a professional with my kind of background and experience. An interview with his management group was essential. I wore my shoes for the first time in about four months. My office clothes and suits were found hanging in my cupboard again. I remember my knees were shaking the first day I stepped into the office. It was a totally different world from the one I had become used to. Since my diagnosis, my outside world had revolved around visits to the hospital or walks in the park. Sometimes a rare drive around the city in the car, with all windows fully closed so as to protect me from the Delhi pollution. And now I was sitting in my very own office. Three times a day for about three hours each time. It was a part-time consultancy. It felt nice. No, it felt great.

I must have been one of the few cancer patients in India who had managed to find a job while they were undergoing treatment. I had been warned that cancer patients were not looked upon very kindly by the corporate world. Their needs varied from day to day. As did their health. And given a chance most Indian companies would not like to have to deal with such unpredictable situations. They would rather that the patient took long leave for treatment. There were no laws in the country that protected cancer patients from prejudices and unfair practices. They did not possess equal rights like they might in the developed western world. They were discriminated against.

Even my oncologist noticed a quickening in my step when I met her for the first time after I had started to work. She commented on my changed attire. My jacket and tie. I even attended office straight after 160 mg. of Taxotere was administered during my fourth cycle. However, in the end I could not complete the three-month assignment. The cumulative effects of the drugs took their toll. My fifth cycle of chemotherapy led to the worst side effects that I had experienced. I was in and out of hospital most of the time. My working days were over.

Objectives and priorities have their own way of adjusting with the situation and the circumstances. Like the day I was all ready for work. But instead of reaching the office, I had to be rushed to hospital as a result of extremely low blood counts. In critical moments, we find it easier to define and relate to our priorities, to what we are up against and to what we must accomplish. And more often than not perseverance pays. However, ask anyone, especially those who have no health complications, what they want from life and what their goals are. In most cases their replies would seem trivial. Most of the spontaneous replies would include promotions at work. Or a fancy new car. An exotic holiday. They would never think of living life fuller. Longer. Or they would need to get their thoughts in order before they are able to come up with some meaningful goals. Yet the same people, if diagnosed as cancer patients, would be able to list a hundred things they want to achieve. A sense of urgency suddenly enters their lives. Time and space acquire a new dimension. A new meaning. And within the long list of things that have to be achieved, they start prioritizing. Life takes a new twist and turn. Days are more organized. Every moment spent, every additional breath taken has value. So much joy. So much hope. It is the 'cancer crisis' that suddenly changes the future ahead.

New priorities are not just a response to a crisis situation. They are not just a sudden act of bravery that is often seen during a battle. Whatever is happening in your life is your own doing. Your own karma. Just as it was before the crisis started. Whatever the situation, only you have the power to decide how you want to look at things. Which way you want your head to turn. Prioritizing can be your hidden guiding spirit, your mentor. And it works in its own subtle ways. Each day, without realizing, you set your own priorities. Some people insist on penning down 'things to do'. Others keep diaries to list appointments and tasks to be accomplished. But these become part of an everyday routine. The 'things to be done' are always more important than the listing. Yet only a few realize that if the listing were not done every day, if the objectives were not properly defined, most of those things would be left undone.

Identifying priorities and setting goals, both short-term as well as long-term, play a vital role. They not only focus all energies on a particular path but also add a new meaning and excitement to life as each day passes. It is the short-term goals that are more important. Focusing on them, achieving them, winning in the short-term brings the mind and body together, sharpens your skills, hardens your resolve. The winning habit is critical, since it uplifts you. It builds your inner strength for the ultimate goal. It makes you believe that even your long-term goals are as easily achievable. Don't be too concerned with the end result. That will take care of itself in due course at the right moment. If you concentrate too much on the end result, you can falter in your path. Don't keep wondering what stage you are at. The beginning of your arduous journey. Or the middle. Or near the final goal. At whichever stage you might be that is the place for you to be at that moment in time and space. Whether it feels comfortable or uncomfortable. Whether it is a happy state to be in. Or sad. Never brood over how long it would take or how much further you have to travel to achieve your ultimate goal. Concentrate your energies on the tasks at hand. Think about winning. Ensure that the goals that you have set for yourself for the moment are being achieved. Each achievement adds to your determination to win the final war.

*The Prophet said, "When you lay one finger
over an eye, you see the world without the sun.
One fingertip hides the moon—
and this is a symbol of God's covering—
the whole world may be hidden from view
by a single point,
and the sun may be eclipsed by a splinter."
Close your lips and gaze on the sea within you:
God made the sea subject to man.*

Jelaluddin Rumi in the *Mathnawi*, I, 3555-8

BATTLE PLAN 6
VISUALIZING YOUR WAY TO HEALTH

Nearly six months had passed since my war against cancer began. In this period, I had fought and won many battles, emerged victorious in many of the skirmishes. Every three weeks I had religiously spent at least two days in hospital to undergo over 15 hours of treatment. Two sessions of chemotherapy each time, one that also required about six hours of hydration before and after the drug flowed into my system. A few hours before the sixth and final cycle of chemotherapy began the doctors decided to change one of the drugs. At the end of the fifth cycle, I had developed some side effects that were believed to have been caused by Cisplatin. There had been some hearing loss and some early signs of neuropathy. But luckily the damage had been noticed at a very early stage and given time, could be reversed. Cisplatin was being replaced by another drug from the same family, Carboplatin.

Right from the very beginning, I had guided the path the drugs had taken in my system. I had visualized each drop, each molecule of the chemotherapy drugs. Combined they formed an army of many trillions of fighting-fit soldiers. They entered through the chemo-port on the left side of my chest, were welcomed into my blood stream, and traveled through the heart to the right side of my lungs. Here they had stayed, unloaded their ammunition, and fought the enemy. Ensured that the enemy was being destroyed. Gradually, in a planned and organized manner. Now there was a change in the battle plan. A new group of soldiers had taken over. A surprise awaited the enemy. My role became that much more critical. I had to ensure that all my forces were properly guided to the war zone. And that they succeeded in the final assault. The enemy within had to be vanquished.

Guiding the path of the chemotherapy drugs during each cycle and visualizing the healing taking place in the body leads to a greater understanding of how the war is being won. A vast army of white blood cells. Each armed with the anti-cancer drugs. Each strong and aggressive. Each ready for battle. Each destroying the weak and disorganized cancer cells. Flushing them out of the system, through the liver and the kidneys. Eliminating them finally through the urine and the stool. The shrinking tumor as each battle progresses, till it finally disappears. With a minimum of damage to the normal cells. A simple battle plan. Vividly pictured and stored and saved in the memory forever. Repeated in similar or marginally different forms in each chemotherapy cycle.

Most times the war zone was overflowing with casualties. The after effects of each battle. Felt in terms of fatigue. Nausea and diarrhea. A complete destruction of the hair follicles right at the beginning that resulted in my losing all my hair. The enemy within was creating new allies and with their help opening up new battle fronts. There was no end to the post-battle repair that needed to be undertaken. And as the drugs were administered to fight on these additional fronts, their path was guided to ensure quick victory in these skirmishes.

Visualization of the destruction of the cancer cells need not necessarily be restricted to fighting a war. The shrinking of the tumor can be pictured in many ways. Like a big fish, the white blood cells powered with the chemotherapy drugs, eating the small fish, the weak and disorganized cancer cells. Or like an overflowing river, gushing through the colony of the cancer cells, creating destruction and havoc, carrying the dead cancer cells as it flows out of the system. At one stage I remember, I pictured the cancer cells as small, black and ugly rats moving haphazardly in my lungs and the chemotherapy drugs like rat poison left in their path. Cancer cells behave like small boats out in the middle of the ocean amidst a bad storm. Or like objects in the path of an avalanche or a hurricane, in full cry and fury, unmindful of the destruction caused. The drugs are like pesticides being sprayed to save the crops. In whichever manner or form the drugs are visualized, havoc and destruction certainly play an important part in the entire process. The drugs not only destroy the cancer cells; they affect all cells in the body, even the good cells that multiply at a fast rate. The drugs cannot differentiate between the bad cells and the good cells. However, it is essential that in the entire visualization process, the images are focused on the destruction of the cancer cells with minimum damage to the good, normal cells. And that the latter are rebuilt as soon as they are destroyed.

How do you, as a cancer patient, benefit from this visualization? For one, you understand how your treatment is working. You begin to participate in improving your health. Being an active participant in your health helps you understand your condition better. It builds on your internal resources to fight the disease. It helps you to increase your belief in your self. Belief that you can and will eventually win.

As the treatment progresses, you gain confidence and can actually feel the tumor shrinking. And the cancer cells being flushed out. This enhances the whole process of self-realization and self-discovery. It brings the mind and body together since mental images of the various activities inside the body are being conjured up at all times.

Mental imagery also helps in the reduction of fear, anxiety and anger you may feel towards your cancer as well as the treatment. Fear arises from the belief that you are not in control and that the fast-growing cancer cells are causing further deterioration in the body. The images generated visualize the orderly destruction of the weak and disorganized cancer cells and remove any negativity that may exist. They highlight and enhance your role in regaining your health. They strengthen the will to live. They help you communicate with your subconscious, reaching out to all parts of your mind and body. And most importantly they keep the mind active, not allowing it to become weak as a result of the side effects of the disease and the treatment.

Mental imagery is not new in our lives. We have been conjuring up various images in our minds since childhood. As little children we have imagined for days before our birthday all the wonderful gifts we would receive. Or before Christmas. A 70 mm cinematic picturisation of the Jack and the Beanstalk story as it was repeated again and again at bedtime. At other times we have visualized the joys of winning. The 100-metre dash or a cricket match. Or excelling in academics or our career. As we grew older, we day dreamt, attempted to draw pictures in our mind of our future spouses. Of beautiful people. Of film stars and other celebrities that we admired. Images of destinations, of holidays. Long lazy afternoons on the beach. Or trekking in the Himalayas.

Rediscovering nature. Didn't all this give us joy? Give us the courage to overcome moments of despair in our lives? Help us in strengthening our resolve to achieve what we desired? Then why should the visualization of the extermination of unwanted cancer cells from some part of our body be any different?

As cancer patients our mental imagery need not necessarily be restricted to the cancer and the treatment. In order to strengthen our positive attitude, we can visualize all that we would do once the war is over. When we have won. Or even picture what we would do once the worst moments of the side effects of the treatment are over. Positive images can only further your cause. There is, however, a danger. At times you can be overtaken by negative imagery. At moments of great despair when everything around you is not working to your satisfaction. When you are losing your grip on the treatment. Losing control over a length of time can be dangerous. And this normally happens when the mind gets flooded with negative images. Pictures that make you feel that the tumor is not shrinking. Pictures that give you the feeling that you are stuck in deep concentric circles or loops and are not being able to come out of them. Images of sinking deeper and deeper in a large pit of quicksand.

One such set of images that always kept coming back to me was related to the loss of my hair. I had always been extremely proud of my hair. No one in my immediate family, who had crossed the age of 50, had thick black hair on his head the way I did. Neither my brothers. Nor my brothers-in-law. Within a few days of my first chemotherapy cycle, I woke up one morning to find my pillow covered with falling hair. And soon it was all gone. From my head. My body. And most of my beard. In those few days, as and when I ran my fingers through my hair, or used my brush, chunks of it would come out. On my hands and fingers. In the brush. In the beginning I collected all the hair that fell so rapidly. I was most disturbed. Though there was no physical pain involved, the mental torture was killing me. My new bald look made me extremely unhappy. More so each time I stood in front of a mirror. Like Samson, I thought I would lose all my strength. My positive resolve. Even though I knew the hair would all come back after the treatment was over.

Amrita tried to raise my spirits by telling me that baldness suited me. And that more and more people, including many celebrities, were shaving their hair on their heads. Newspaper and magazine pictures of people with bald heads were collected by my children. My friends tried to convince me that this was the latest fashion. The new craze the world over. But nothing helped. For a long period I was extremely depressed about the loss of hair. I felt embarrassed about my baldness. I stopped going out. I refused to meet people. In my moments alone I cried. Today when I look back nothing else caused me as much anguish as my loss of hair. And the fear that it might never come back. That I would be bald for the rest of my life. I thought about a wig. Or a cap to cover my head. I felt naked on my head. It became an obsession. I started to feel cold on my head, even in the middle of the hot Delhi summers. Gradually I accepted my fate.

I remember it took many weeks for me to begin to accept my new look. It started with mental images of the period in my youth when I had long, shoulder-length hair. That was the fashion in the '60s. The decade of the Beatles. Woodstock. Drugs. Anti-Vietnam. Long hair. I began to visualize how I would feel on the day I could brush my hair again. The mental pain and images of my baldness still continued. Their intensity, however, lessened. I had begun to accept the loss of my hair. In more or less the same manner as I had accepted my cancer. The difference was that I had accepted the cancer soon after it was confirmed. The loss of my hair took longer and caused deep mental anguish.

In the entire visualization process, you should not ignore or suppress any mental images. Nor should you attempt to analyze or judge their content. You should simply make a mental note of them and observe them as specific events in your awareness. Paradoxically, these images that come and go in your mind can make you feel less caught up in them and give you a deeper perspective on your reaction to the daily stress and pressures of cancer and its treatment. By observing these images from a distance, as if you were not so deeply involved with them, you can see much more clearly what is actually on your mind. You can see images arise and recede, one into the other. They are just a pictorial expression of your emotions. Your beliefs. Your desires. Your frustrations. At that moment in time and space. You can make a mental note of the contents, the feelings that are associated with them, and your reactions. This will help you gain insight into what drives you. How you see the world and how you see yourself. And provide an insight into your fears and aspirations, which are leading to most of the stress and pressures you are experiencing. The key is not so much what you choose to focus on but the quality of the awareness that you bring to each moment. It is very important that it be more of a silent witnessing, a dispassionate observing, than a running commentary on your inner experiences.

Observing without judging, moment by moment, helps you visualize what is on your mind without editing or censoring it, without intellectualizing or getting lost in your own thinking.

An investigative, discerning observation destroys the true and innermost flow of mental images. As a student of science, I had always believed that the very act of observation changes the true status of what is being observed. The goal is for you to be more aware, more in touch with your own life and with whatever is happening in your mind-body continuum at the time it is happening — that is, in the present moment. If, for instance, you are experiencing a negative image, you should resist the impulse to try and escape the unpleasantness. Instead, you must attempt to see it clearly as it is and accept it because it is already present for that moment. And it will, more often than not, automatically disappear on its own, as you begin to see the positive side of the negative image. Even negativity has its own inherent meanings. It has its own reason to be present at that moment. Acceptance of a negative image does not indicate passivity or resignation. On the contrary, by fully accepting the images that each moment offers, you open yourself to experiencing life much more completely and make it easier for yourself to respond effectively to any situation that confronts you. Even the worst of the side effects of the treatment. Acceptance offers a way to navigate life's ups and downs with grace, with a sense of humor, and perhaps provides some understanding of the big picture, your ultimate goal.

Mental imagery is like the surface of large ocean. There are always waves, sometimes big, sometimes small. The attempt is not to stop the waves so that the water will be flat, peaceful, and tranquil. The stopping of the waves is beyond your control. They are governed by laws that you may or may not understand. You can however harness their energies. You can ride the waves. You can surf. Focus your attention fully on the present moment and be in tune with all the mental images that are being conjured. By being aware, by developing an open mind and a more accepting attitude, the psychological and emotional causes of pain and suffering will get relieved. And with this release, there will be a decrease in the stress and the pressures, removing all the unwanted blocks to the healing that is taking place within.

Negative imagery, more often than not, is a result of the patient's own frustrations. At not being able to achieve what he or she set out to achieve for that moment of time and space. It is most often riddled with stress, tension and even fear. All this arising out of the long period of time that the treatment takes. Or a sudden change in the treatment. Even a slight aberration can lead to drastic shifts in mental images. And once the pendulum has swung it has to be brought back on track as soon as possible. Negative imagery is the result of the stress and tension that has surfaced as a result of the cancer and its treatment. And visualization helps in relieving stress and increasing the sense of self-control. As do yoga, meditation and chanting which can also achieve dramatic results.

Shrava aasan helps in releasing body and muscle tension. Start by lying down comfortably in a darkened room with your eyes shut. Breathe slowly and deeply. As you breathe in, concentrate all your mental and physical energies on your toes and keep repeating in your mind that your toes are becoming relaxed. Move from one toe to the other, and from the toes to the ankles, the calves, and the knees, to all the different parts of the leg so as to relax them in a similar manner. And from one leg to the other, and then to the other parts of the body, concentrating especially on those parts where you had felt greater tension. If you are undergoing medication, you can also concentrate more on those parts that need the treatment. At the same time, visualize your muscles getting relaxed. As you breathe in, tense the muscles that you may be working on, hold your breath for a moment with the muscles remaining tense, and as you breathe out, release the tension, thereby relaxing the muscles. And picture the muscles and the body being relieved of all the tension. Once every part of the body has been covered in this manner, continue to lie still with your eyes closed. Enjoy the feeling of a totally relaxed mind and body. Such a progressive relaxation of the body, along with a mental imagery of the release of tension in each part of the body is an ancient yogic technique. *Shrava* literally means 'dead body' and to be able to reach this state is the ultimate form of the mind-body equilibrium, relaxation of all the muscles, the tension, the stress and the negative imagery that the mind and body might be riddled with.

Meditation, on the other hand, makes use of rhythmic breathing and relies heavily on the conjuring up of mental images. While there are various forms of meditation, listening to audiocassettes of reiki meditation provided me the solace and comfort that I was looking for. Every other day during the treatment, I used to wake up empty and frightened. And to overcome this fear, someone suggested that I practice meditation to further relax my mind and body. I began by focusing attention on the sensation of breath leaving and entering my body. Anything else that entered my mind was like a distraction that I did my utmost to disregard. It was not the easiest thing to accomplish. But over a period of time, this mental imagery of my breathing gave rise to a deep state of calm. I was able to trace the entire path that my breath took inside my body, from the point of entry to all the goodness that it generated till the time it got flushed out eventually.

Each process lasting not for long, but repeating itself at regular intervals without a break, in a manner that only I could identify with. As soon as I was comfortable with this single point focus of my breathing, I was able to visualize scenes of utmost peace and tranquility, of a free flow of joy that I had never experienced. Of my breath flowing freely and naturally as I allowed myself to float and drift and relax in a cosmic sea of life-giving energy or reiki. As this life force energy cleansed and healed the innermost parts of my body, my cancer, I experienced a feeling of becoming lighter and flowing into this energy, as it slowly and steadily engulfed my entire body and mind. I visualized the white light, the violet flame and all their healing vibrations. The meditation providing an experience of a much higher reality and bliss than I had ever experienced before.

Chanting too allows you to focus on the task at hand. In the Hindu way of life, many mantras have been used to bring mind and body into a sharper focus. Each has its own benefits. Each brings its own joy and peace. I found my peace, my tranquility in the Buddhist chant of 'nam-myoho-renge-kyo'. We all have the inherent ability to live with courage, to have fulfilling relationships and to face and surmount our deepest problems. Crucial to the realization of this ability is an inner transformation. We need a way to access our unlimited potential. As we chant 'nam-myoho-renge-kyo', as we visualize the changes that are taking place inside our mind and body, we find unlimited wisdom, courage, hope, confidence and endurance from within ourselves. Instead of fearing or avoiding thinking about the cancer and its treatment, we find the energy to confront it with vigor, confident in our ability to surmount it with our own internal resources. Life is ever changing. The only constant in life is change. At one moment we may feel the courage to win the war against cancer. At the next we can be totally overwhelmed by the simplest of pressures of the cancer treatment. A slight nausea or discomfort. But through steady daily chanting of 'nam-myoho-renge-kyo' we continue to strengthen our resolve.

Mental imagery arises out of our thoughts, our feelings, and our emotions. It can be negative or positive. It can be under our control as long as it originates from our conscious state. The imagery can be used to guide the flow of drugs during the treatment. It can be used to fight cancer, pain or any other side effects of the treatment. It can be used to reduce stress and pressures arising from the treatment or even as a result of any other external influence. It should be allowed all the freedom of free-flow. It needs no observation or detailed analysis.

There are also other forms of imagery that are essentially controlled by the subconscious state. Much has been written about them. And various theories have been propounded to understand them better. They are open for analysis, and their meanings are often sought. At most times they are beyond our control. And very often memory lapses occur and they are readily forgotten. These include dreams and daydreams, generated as a result of some unexplained chemistry in our mind and body equilibrium.

Dreams are nothing but a continuation of our mental imagery in sleep. During the day, the mind-body continuum leads to a large diversity of mental images, visual manifestations of pain, stress, joy, expectations, intent, love, etc. These images get extended in a somewhat similar manner at night when we sleep. If we look more closely into our dreams, and try to analyze them, we realize the significance of the waking mental images. Dreams can be such that they represent the fulfillment of our deepest desires and wishes; and others in which this fulfillment is unrecognizable and often concealed by every available means. There are also painful dreams that are considered to be punishment dreams. The recognition and analysis of dreams makes us realize that the power behind the dream is governed by the subconscious. Every dream shows in its content a connection with a recent waking impression, often similar to our mental imagery. Throughout the night the subconscious is working overtime while the conscious state is oriented to the mind and body being asleep. The progress of the residual images from the waking activity of the mind is now being governed by the subconscious, which is in full control even when deeper and deeper sleep gets induced. And since the process of waking up requires time, it is during this period that we remember most of the visual images that transpire in our dreams. The final pictures of the dream are often so vivid that they force us to awaken: in reality they are so vivid only because when they appear we are already very near waking.

There is a hairline difference between mental imagery that we experience in our waking moments and the picture sequences generated in our dreams. The beginning of a dream is the beginning of the wakening process and, more often than not, the dream is an extension of the mental images that the thought processes conjure up during the waking day. At most times we try and analyze our dreams whenever we can remember the visual sequences that transpired when we were dreaming. We talk about them to others. Some believe that what we dream would at some stage actually happen in the real world or had happened in the past. At times we dream all night, but cannot remember any of the images we dreamt. At other occasions, we perceive that something has been dreamt if we are suddenly roused from a deep sleep. There are greater chances of recall of those dreams that are capable of waking us in the midst of our sleep. Dreams, even if they interrupt our sleep several times a night, still remain compatible with sleep. We wake up for a moment, and often immediately fall asleep again. Thinking ahead, making resolutions, visualizing and sketching attempted solutions that can then perhaps be realized at some stage in our lives, nightmares — these and many more images are all functions of the subconscious, all mental imagery that gets conjured up in our sleep. And those dreams that we can remember provide us a true insight to our subconscious.

On the other hand, daydreaming makes use of spontaneous mental imagery in visualizing personal experiences of the past or of the future. It is often also viewed as a useless distraction from the task at hand. Daydreaming is all about the process of creativity in generating new and useful images in any specific situation. It's about how emotions can be regulated at any moment in time and space. For example, when your oncologist informs you that your tumor has shrunk, different images flash in your mind and you may or may not sink into a daydream. If you do, then more often than not, daydreaming enables you to visualize all that you would accomplish once your war against cancer is over. Many differing daydream sequences are possible depending on your creative energies. Starting with mental images of winning the war, you may move on to daydreaming about going out for lunch with your favourite movie star or a family holiday at an exotic beach resort. Or some other dream sequence that is equally pleasant and has been on your mind. One sequence leads to another, till you wake up from a somewhat sleepy state. Your emotional state triggers the daydreams and daydreams modify the existing emotions and trigger new emotions, which trigger new daydreams, and so on. Daydreams usually lead to or are a result of positive and pleasant emotions, though painful ones cannot be ruled out. Their images have a far greater influence on the entire healing process and your thoughts and emotions than the mental images that you may conjure up through your conscious state during the moments you are fully awake. They are far more powerful and can get recalled either instantly or later through analogies. The lunch with the movie star may get recalled while watching a movie in which the star plays a major role and the beach resort while reading a travel magazine or while making a holiday plan. And so on.

We are all a part of a huge universe of energy that generates its own visions, its own pictures, and its own ideas. And we can understand and accept this to whatever depth we are able. This ocean of infinite images, the intricate manner of their inter-connectivity is fascinating, but far too complex for our understanding. What we do know is that all our mental images, irrespective of their form, are inspired and generated from our conscious state and eventually get implanted in the mind and body equilibrium. The development of images, their scrutiny and their examination, generates confidence as more and more experiences and images are shared. Even the free-flowing mental images, generated by our conscious state and with the absence of any form of detailed analysis, deepen our understanding, as more and more images are experienced. Mental images are windows that open into higher dimensions of the mind. A cone can

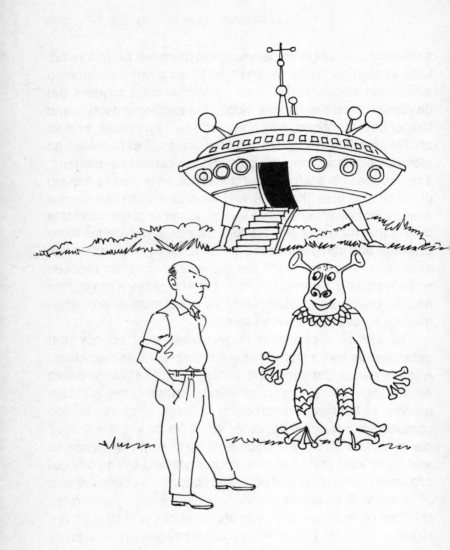

*"I looked just like you before I started
my chemotherapy."*

yield different two-dimensional shapes, even circles or ellipses, when cut on its cross-section and yet intrinsically, it still remains a cone. Reality is something that changes according to the manner in which it is observed. All images are unified at some level. And all images are but facets of our inner being. In probing the other we always come back with images of ourselves. In probing ourselves we return with images of the other. In the phenomenon of being, we are merely privileged observers of a relationship between the conscious and the subconscious states. How this relationship came to be, and what its limitations are, we cannot know until we gain access to all the mental imagery that is possible.

It is not subject to the will of any individual. It has its own will and an understanding that is more sophisticated than any one of us who reaps its benefits. It has a plan, glimpsed by us only as vision. And in a manner, governed by laws that are unknown to humankind, it drives us closer to our ultimate goal. A dream that we, as cancer patients, together share. A visual sequence that is critical to our participation in our treatment. Pictures that provide an understanding of our inner self and the healing process within. After all, a picture is worth more than a thousand words.

*The doctor of the future will give no medicine
but will interest his patients in the care of the
human frame,
in diet, and in the cause and prevention of disease....
The physician of tomorrow will be the nutritionist of today.*

Thomas Edison

BATTLE PLAN 7
CONTROLLING YOUR DIET

Food. Glorious food. Mouth-watering delicacies. All that I had always wanted to eat. At each meal. Between meals. They were all there, cooked, ready to eat, especially for me. Only what I liked mattered. Only my favourite foods were brought before me. I was badly pampered. Yet for the few days after each chemotherapy cycle my appetite vanished. Those were the days when I had to build on my reserves. Those were the days the different parameters of my blood reduced to alarmingly low levels. And apart from the medication that I was being given to bring them back to normal, I was also supposed to eat well so that they improved naturally with the nourishment from the food. But the side effects of the treatment prevented this from happening.

Small quantities. Consumed every hour. Even that did not help. The foul taste in the mouth as a result of the drugs. I had no idea that I would ever find food so disgusting. Devoid of taste. Flavours that I could not recognize. Food full of love and care. Cooked by Amrita. For the first few days I was not able to retain the food that I consumed. After that the heavy doses of medication to control the nausea began to take effect. But not before I had lost a few kilograms of weight, some of which were regained before the next chemotherapy cycle started.

Exercise was another point of failure during that period. I just could not get myself to go for my daily exercise; something that my oncologist had said was absolutely essential. Instead of walking for about 20 kilometers a week, I was able to complete less that half of what my oncologist had advised. I knew I was letting down my mind and body. But while the intent was there, the motivation was totally missing.

In the four months that have elapsed, I have read a great deal about how diet and nutrition can help in controlling cancer. The human system is built from, repaired by and energized with substances in our diet. You are what you eat, what you think and what you do. Balanced nutrition and a proper diet succeed in re-establishing the metabolic balance to fight cancer. Many programs have been developed, tried and tested the world over. Pure vegetarian diet. High protein diet. Seafood. Fruits and juices. Fat-free food. And many more. In the end, I came to the conclusion that the best diet to follow is the one that you, the cancer patient, are the most comfortable with. Obviously nourishment is extremely important. But even more important is what you can easily digest. Especially when the side effects of chemotherapy kill your appetite. You can eat only small quantities at a time, so you end up eating more frequently, instead of the standard three meals a day.

Knowledge about diet and nutrition in relation to cancer and their potential to lower the risk of cancer incidence does not necessarily translate to reduction of cancer. Changes in lifestyle are also imperative. People often resist such changes, as is evident from the fact that many continue to smoke, even when they know that a strong link exists between smoking and cancer. When people are diagnosed as patients of cancer, or for that matter any other life-threatening disease, their lives change dramatically. In the way they react to their environment. Their food habits. And much more. Life is never the same again for them. I too experienced such a transformation. Prior to my cancer diagnosis, I had enjoyed all the benefits and comforts of so-called 'good living'. Totally unconcerned about the food I ate. The number of cigarettes I smoked. Consumption of alcohol. Irregular sleep times. Little or no exercise. But this still did not make me the ideal candidate for cancer. Except maybe for the smoking habit. There were others around me who lived more or less similar lifestyles. Some had even more 'degenerate' lifestyles than mine. Then there were those whose lifestyles were very 'healthy'. But amongst all of us, I was the one selected to carry the cancer torch. From within my family and my friends.

Today, after nearly four months of treatment, I sometimes feel that I should have made changes in my life much earlier. But would that have prevented my cancer? My karma? It is not that I have deep regrets about the way I had lived earlier. It was the ideal way to be at that moment in time and space. But today, things have changed. A transformation has taken place and a new being has taken over. Cancer has altered the way I look, feel and react to everything in my environment. I have been born again at the age of 50.

For many people, changes are extremely difficult to accept, and living healthier lives impossible. Healthy living involves eating well, being active and feeling good about oneself. Healthy living helps to achieve a healthy weight in a positive and safe way. A healthy body weight is the weight at which you will feel fit and flexible; feel energetic. Regular physical activity combined with healthy eating, not dieting, is the best formula for achieving and maintaining a healthy weight, a healthy mind and body, leading to healthy living.

A change in any form requires a lot of effort. Under normal circumstances it is difficult to bring about changes in lifestyle. There are too many pressures. Like giving up the smoking habit is impossible because of one silly and stupid reason or the other. It's when faced with a crisis that change in some form is easier to accept. More so a change in eating habits. In matters of food habits, not only do tastes have to change, but also a lot of creative thinking and planning are necessary. Meal planning has a new meaning. A new dimension. A new daily shopping list is required. Different kinds of foods have to be bought. Different sections of the supermarkets have to be visited. The manner in which food is prepared has to be altered. The body has to get used to the absence of the earlier foods that may no longer be a part of the new diet. Imagine a shift from a non-vegetarian diet to one that is purely vegetarian. New foods enter the kitchen. And if some members of the family are not willing to co-operate in the change, different sets of meals have to be prepared.

Recent studies indicate that improper diet and food habits can lead to cancer. The Japanese have one of the lowest rates of cancer prevalence in the world. Typically their diet comprises rice, vegetables and seafood. However, as and when some of them migrate to America, even as close to their homeland as Hawaii, they begin to accept the American way of life. And to a great extent, their diet changes to fat-rich foods including large helpings of steak, red meats and junk foods. Incidence of cancer amongst the Japanese living in America is more or less the same as the American average, which is considered to be the highest in the world. And the change in diet is the one major factor that has contributed to this higher risk of cancer. Today, most cancers can be prevented. An estimated 60% to 70% of cancers are preventable through simple changes in diet and lifestyle. Eating right, plus staying physically active and maintaining a healthy weight, can cut cancer risk by 30% to 40%. Recommended dietary choices, coupled with not smoking, have the potential to reduce cancer risk by 60% to 70%. This would mean that in America alone, as many as 375,000 cases of cancer, at the current rate of cancer prevalence, can be prevented each year through healthy living practices.

What are these healthy practices? In dietary terms, choosing a predominantly plant-based diet, rich in a variety of vegetables and fruits, pulses and a minimum of processed starchy staple foods. Eating 400-800 grams daily of a variety of vegetables and fruits, all year round, together with 600-800 grams of a variety of cereals, pulses, roots, tubers and plantains. Avoiding processed foods and limiting the consumption of refined sugar. Avoid being underweight or overweight and limit weight gain during adulthood to less than 5kg. Intake of red meat should be minimum and less than 80 grams daily. Fish and chicken are preferable to red meat. Avoid fatty foods, particularly those of animal origin. Do not eat charred food. For meat and fish eaters, avoid burning of meat and avoid grilled meat and fish; or cured and smoked meats. Choose modest amounts of appropriate vegetable oils. Limit consumption of salted foods and use of cooking and table salt. Use herbs and spices to season foods. Do not eat food that, as a result of prolonged storage at ambient temperatures, is liable to contamination with mycotoxins. Unregulated levels of additives, contaminants and other residues can be a health hazard. If occupational activity is low or moderate, take an hour's brisk walk or similar exercise daily, and also exercise vigorously for a total of at least an hour every week. Alcohol consumption is not recommended, and if consumed, limit alcoholic drinks to less than two drinks a day for men and one for women. And above, all do not smoke or chew tobacco.

People who have more fiber and less fat in their diet have a lower incidence of certain types of cancers. Also, a positive link has been found between consumption of vegetables that are fiber-rich, and the reduction of risk of certain types of cancer. In addition to dietary fiber, vegetables offer vitamins and minerals as natural 'plant chemicals' that work together to lower cancer risk. Dietary fiber helps maintain a steady level in blood sugar and insulin; keeps the appetite satisfied longer; dilutes harmful substances, and speeds their elimination. Animal products like meat, cheese and eggs contain no fiber. And only plant foods like fruits, vegetables, whole grains, beans, nuts and seeds, provide the fiber necessary for good health. Some vegetables, fruits and grain products are higher in fiber than others. For example, a half-cup of cooked carrots has four times as much fiber as a cup of raw spinach. A medium baked potato contains more fiber than a half-cup of cooked brown rice. Whole wheat bread has twice as much fiber as white bread. No matter what specific foods are selected, eating a variety of fruits, vegetables, grains and beans ensures the daily intake of fiber and the nutrients that are critical to lowering cancer risk.

Not only do vegetables provide protection against cancer, they are also essential for a healthy diet. Vegetables with the highest anti-cancer activity include garlic, cabbage, soybeans, ginger and carrots. Vegetables with modest anti-cancer activity include onions, broccoli, Brussels sprouts, cauliflower, tomato and peppers. There are many reasons why there is so much support and emphasis being laid on a daily diet that is rich in fruits and vegetables. These foods are major sources of vitamins, minerals, biochemical compounds, and fiber-ingredients that can help reduce the cancer risk. Moreover, eating enough fruits and vegetables means a person is likely to eat proportionately less fatty and high-calorie foods. Fruits and vegetables are chemically very complex, and contain many bio-chemicals that can contribute to reducing the risk of cancer.

A low-fat diet can also reduce the overall cancer risk. The risk of some kinds of cancer may be more as a result of a high-fat diet than other kinds of cancer. Also, since fat can be of many kinds, some forms have different effects on cancer risk than others. Fats may be saturated or unsaturated, and there are different kinds of saturated and unsaturated fats. Also, in a high-fat diet, it is sometimes hard to distinguish whether the risk is due to the fat present or to the diet being high in calories. The amount of fat you eat will vary from day to day. Some meals and some days will be higher in fat. That's okay. Even high fat meals can be in keeping with healthy eating, as long as these meals are balanced with lower fat meals. It is the average intake of fat over the course of weeks and months that is important, not the fat content of every food and meal eaten.

Food is composed of a vast number of different chemical ingredients, including some components that tend to increase cancer risk. Some of these chemicals (carcinogens) are natural ingredients of the diet and may be unavoidable. Other carcinogens are the result of contaminants, or result from the way food is prepared (charcoal cooked, broiled or smoked foods). Not only are different kinds of foods necessary in the diet but they must be prepared in different ways; mix and match foods in ways that haven't been tried before to avoid eating the same old things, week in and week out. Variety is important because it increases the chances of getting all of the nutrients needed for good health, in the right amounts. Variety also stacks the diet with protective factors that may disarm the would-be cancer causing substances.

The onslaught of cancer is a likely sign that the liver may have been functioning poorly for sometime. The liver is a vital ally to the immune system in the war on cancer and protects the body by removing toxic substances from the bloodstream that might lead to cancer. The longer the toxic wastes stay in the bloodstream, the greater are the chances of the poisons being reabsorbed. And this can be disastrous. It's like removing the garbage every morning, letting it rot for sometime, and then bringing it back for dinner. Not only does the liver have to work overtime as a result of the re-entry of the pollutants in the system, the blood delivers these poisons throughout the body, where they have the opportunity to create further damage. For a healthy body, a thorough cleansing of the liver, the gall bladder and the colon is essential through regular bowel movements. There are greater chances of cancer developing in a body that has lost the normal functions as a consequence of a chronic daily poisoning, accumulated over time, especially in the liver.

Nutrition is a low-cost, non-toxic component in the overall war against cancer. An aggressive nutrition program in your daily battle-plan is critical since it avoids malnutrition that can result from either the cancer or the treatment. It also reduces the toxicity of the medical therapy and helps the treatment become more selectively toxic to the cancer cells. It stimulates the immune functions and selectively starves the tumor. And finally it acts as a defense mechanism and improves the performance and outcome of the drugs. In order to lower the side effects of the treatment, there are many ways to increase food intake and improve nutrition. And also to ensure that you continue eating as well as you can when the treatment or illness is resulting in the worst of its side effects. Long-term treatment, especially chemotherapy, may necessitate changes in the diet so as to help in coping with the side effects and rebuilding of strength and immunity. Each chemotherapy drug gives rise to different side effects. So eventually, you have to find what works best for you.

Good nutrition is even more important for people with cancer. Patients who eat well during their treatment are able to cope better with the side effects of treatment. Patients who eat well may be able to handle higher doses of certain treatments. A healthy diet helps keep up your strength, prevents body tissues from breaking down, and rebuilds tissues that the cancer treatment may harm. When you are unable to eat enough food or the right kind of food, your body uses stored nutrients as a source of energy. And as a result, your natural defenses, which have already been weakened with cancer, get weaker and your body cannot fight infection as well. Your defense system is especially important to you now, because cancer patients are often at risk of getting an infection. A good rule to follow is to eat a variety of different foods every day. No one food or group of foods contains all of the nutrients you need and only a variety of foods can meet your requirements. During certain days, you may probably need more calories and more high-protein foods, such as meats and dairy products. On other days, you may need to cut back on high-fiber foods for a while, such as vegetables, fruits, cereals, and whole grains, if your treatment is causing diarrhea. Your oncologist may also recommend additional commercial nutrition supplements to make sure you get enough protein, calories, and other nutrients during treatment.

Pay attention to the changing needs of your body. As each battle is fought and won. As the treatment progresses. And as and when you are overcome by the side effects of the treatment. If nausea, the most common side effect of the treatment, makes certain foods unappealing, then eat more of the foods you find easier to handle. Sometimes changing the form of a food will make it more appetizing and help you eat better. It is important to keep trying new things. Anything you eat will be a plus in getting enough calories to maintain your weight. It is important that you avoid uncooked and raw fruits and vegetables since they can lead to infection. Also it is essential that all food is cooked in a clean and hygienic manner.

The methods of treating cancer, viz. surgery, radiation therapy and chemotherapy, are very powerful. And the drugs and medication used are some of the strongest known to humankind. Although most of these treatments target the cancer cells in the body, they also damage the normal and healthy cells. And this is what produces the unpleasant side effects that cause the eating problems. The side effects of cancer treatment vary from patient to patient. The part of the body being treated, the length of treatment, and the dose of treatment and the drugs used also determine whether the side effects will occur. Cancer treatment can also affect your eating in another way. Stress, worry or fear of cancer or the treatment can lead to eating problems. Losing your appetite and nausea are two normal responses to feeling nervous or fearful. Such problems should last only a short time. Don't be afraid to give food a chance. Not everyone has problems with eating during cancer treatment. Even those who have eating problems have days when eating is a pleasure. Always share your needs and concerns with your family particularly those who plan and prepare the meals for you. Let them know how much you appreciate their support and efforts as you work towards overcoming eating problems.

Thus far I have completed four of my six cycles of chemotherapy. The side effects, except for the persistent nausea that prevailed for at least five to six days each time, varied each time. Sometimes the nausea would lead to vomiting. During certain cycles I suffered from diarrhea. In others, I was constipated. I remember in my first cycle I went through both in a span of four days, maybe as a consequence of the medication I was given to control the initial diarrhea. As a result of these side effects, my intake of food during the first few days after the administration of the chemotherapy drugs was extremely poor. And this just added to my other problems caused by the side effects of the drugs. The significant parameters of my blood usually hovered around the lower permissible levels. Sometimes they went below the lower limits. I was beginning to get black-outs while standing or walking. Was this the result of weakness arising out of poor food intake? Or were these the side effects of the drugs? My oncologist said it was a bit of both. Efforts were made to bring the parameters of my blood within the normal acceptable limits. A series of injections. Blood transfusions. Iron supplements. Iron-rich foods. And more. Medication to control the other side effects.

Nausea, with or without vomiting, is a common side effect of surgery, chemotherapy, and radiation therapy. Cancer itself, or the treatment, or even other conditions unrelated to your cancer or treatment, may cause nausea. Whatever the cause, nausea prevents you from getting enough food and the much-needed nutrients. Most cancer treatments lead to nausea and medication is provided to help reduce it. In order to ensure that your intake of food is not reduced in any manner, you can eat toast, yogurt, skinned chicken (baked or broiled, not fried), fruits and vegetables that are soft or bland, clear liquids (sipped slowly), etc. Avoid eating fatty, greasy, fried, spicy or hot food with strong odors, and sweets. Avoid eating in a room that's stuffy, too warm, or has cooking odors that might disagree with you. Drink fewer liquids with meals since drinking liquids can cause a full, bloated feeling. Drink or sip liquids throughout the day, except at mealtimes. Drink beverages cool or chilled. Eat foods at room temperature or cooler; hot foods may add to nausea. Don't force yourself to eat your favorite foods when you feel nauseated since this may lead to a permanent dislike of those foods. Rest after meals, because hectic activity can slow down digestion. Wear loose-fitting clothes. Avoid eating for one to two hours before treatment, so as to prevent nausea during the radiation therapy or chemotherapy. Make a note of when your nausea occurs and what it is most often caused by. It could be a specific food, event, or even something in the environment.

Vomiting may follow nausea and may be brought on by the treatment, or food odours, or gas in the stomach or the bowel. With some patients, certain surroundings, such as the hospital, may lead to vomiting. If vomiting is severe or lasts for more than a few days, contact your oncologist. Very often, if you can control nausea, you can prevent vomiting. At times, though, you may not be able to prevent either nausea or vomiting. Do not drink or eat until you have the vomiting under control. Once you have controlled the vomiting, try small amounts of clear liquids. And keep increasing the quantity and the frequency of consumption. When you are able to retain clear liquids, try a full-liquid diet. Continue taking small amounts as often as you can retain them. And gradually work up to your regular diet.

Diarrhea may have several causes, including chemotherapy, radiation therapy, infection, food sensitivity and emotional upset. Long-term or severe diarrhea may cause other problems. During diarrhea, food passes quickly through the bowel before the body absorbs enough vitamins, minerals, and water. This may cause dehydration and increase the risk of infection. Take the advice of your oncologist if the diarrhea is severe or lasts for more than a couple of days. Drink plenty of liquids during the day. Drinking fluids is important because your body may not get enough water when you have diarrhea. Eat small amounts of food throughout the day instead of three large meals. Eat foods and drink liquids that contain salt and potassium. These minerals are often lost during diarrhea. Foods high in potassium that don't cause diarrhea include bananas, peach, and boiled or mashed potatoes. You can also try to eat other nutritious low-fiber foods like yogurt, curds, rice, skinned chicken or fish (boiled or baked, not fried), cottage cheese, etc. Eliminate greasy, fatty, or fried foods, raw vegetables and fruits; high-fiber vegetables; and strong spices. Avoid very hot or very cold foods and beverages. Do not consume foods and beverages that contain caffeine, including coffee, strong tea, sodas, and chocolate. Be careful when using milk and milk products because diarrhea may be caused by lactose intolerance. After a sudden, short-term attack of diarrhea, try a liquid diet during the first 12 to 14 hours. This will let the bowel rest while replacing the important body fluids lost.

Some anti-cancer drugs and other drugs, such as pain-killers, may cause constipation. This can also occur if your diet lacks fluid or fiber or if you have been bedridden. Drink plenty of liquids, at least eight 8-ounce glasses every day. This will help to keep your stools soft. Take a hot drink about half an hour before your usual time for a bowel movement. Eat high-fiber foods. Exercise everyday. Consult your oncologist about the amount and type of exercise that is right for you. And before taking any laxatives or stool softeners always consult your oncologist.

Loss of appetite or poor appetite is one of the most common problems that occur with cancer and its treatment. Many things affect appetite, including nausea, vomiting and being upset or depressed about having cancer. If you have these feelings, whether physical or emotional, you may not be interested in eating at most times. Make your meal times more relaxed so that you feel more like eating. Stay calm, especially at meal times. Don't hurry your meals. Try changing the time, place, and environment of meals. Set a colorful table. Listen to soft music while eating. Eat with others or watch your favorite TV program while you eat. Eat whenever you are hungry. You do not need to eat just three main meals a day. Several small meals throughout the day may be even better. Add variety to your menu. Eat food often during the day, even at bedtime. Always have healthy snacks handy. Taking just a few bites of the right foods or sips of the right liquids every hour or so can help you get more protein and calories.

Mouth sores, tender gums, and a sore throat often result from radiation therapy, anti-cancer drugs, and infection. If you have a sore mouth or gums, consult your oncologist to be sure the soreness is a side effect of the treatment and not an unrelated dental problem. Your oncologist may be able to give you medicine that will control mouth and throat pain. There are certain foods that will irritate an already tender mouth and make chewing and swallowing difficult. By carefully choosing the foods you eat and by taking good care of your mouth, you can usually make eating easier. Try soft foods that are easy to chew and swallow, such as milkshakes, stewed fruits, mashed potatoes, macaroni, custards, puddings, gelatin, cooked cereals, pureed or mashed vegetables, and so on. Avoid foods like citrus fruits or juice, spicy or salty foods, rough, coarse, or dry foods such as raw vegetables, toast, etc. that can irritate your mouth. Food should be cooked until it is soft and tender and cut into small pieces. Mix food with butter, thin gravies, and sauces to make it easier to swallow. A blender or food processor to puree your food may be a better idea. Use a straw to drink liquids. Try foods cold or at room temperature. Hot and warm foods can irritate a tender mouth and throat. If swallowing is hard, tilting your head back or moving it forward may help. If heartburn is a problem, try sitting up or standing for about an hour after eating. Rinse your mouth with water often to remove food and bacteria and to promote healing.

Your sense of taste or smell may change during your cancer treatment. Foods can acquire a bitter or metallic taste, especially meat or other high-protein foods, and many foods may have less or no taste. Chemotherapy, radiation therapy, or the cancer itself may cause these problems. There is no way to improve the flavor or smell of food because each person is affected differently by cancer and the treatment. However, it helps to choose and prepare foods that look and smell good to *you*. If red meat tastes or smells strange, eat chicken or fish that doesn't have a strong smell. In any case red meats should be avoided as much as possible. Improve the flavor of meat, chicken, or fish by marinating in sweet fruit juices, wine, dressing, or a sauce. Or by using small amounts of flavours or seasonings. Try other foods that may have a different taste or might taste better and also provide the needed protein and calories. Serve food at room temperature. Use, or stop the use of onions, garlic and ginger to add or remove the flavour to vegetables. Stay away from foods that may cause an unpleasant taste.

Chemotherapy and radiation therapy in the head or neck area can reduce the flow of saliva and often cause a dry mouth. When this happens, foods are harder to chew and swallow. A dry mouth can change the way food tastes. Try very sweet foods and beverages such as lemonade. These foods may help your mouth produce more saliva. Suck on sweets or chew gum. These again can help produce more saliva. Use soft and pureed foods, which may be easier to swallow. Keep your lips moist with lip moisturizers. Eat foods with sauces, gravies, and dressings to make them moist and easier to swallow. Have a sip of water every few minutes to help you swallow and talk more easily.

Your body needs both rest and nourishment during and after the treatment for cancer. A regular intake of vitamins and minerals helps in rebuilding the healthy cells that get destroyed by the treatment. And also reinforces the body's own protective systems. Cancer is a degenerative disease, the treatment can be effective and the war can be won only by bringing back the laws that govern both the mind and the body. And by ensuring that all the millions of cells in the body follow the rules. All the haphazard cancer cells are flushed out. It is not just enough to treat the symptoms or treat the cancer, but the reactions and functions of the body and the mind also have to be restored. The treatment and cure and the final victory are an enormous rebuilding task. The reconstruction of the healthy cells that were destroyed in the many battles fought. The rejuvenation of the mind and the body. And the spirit. The overcoming of the mental and emotional trauma. And the physical shock the body has experienced in the long drawn out struggle.

Most of the vitamins and minerals that are recommended during the treatment do not cure cancer. But they are critical for the rebuilding process. The nutrition absorbed by the body from our diet more often than not has to be supplemented with added vitamins and minerals. Vitamin A is a prime component of a strong immune system and stimulates the lymphocytes to fight cancer. It is also the key to cell differentiation and an excellent antioxidant. The latter property helps in fighting the free radicals in the body that cause cancer. Vitamin B-complex works to enhance and stimulate the immune system and inhibits the growth of cancer cells and tumors. Vitamin C is one of the most potent antioxidants and its absence or reduced level increases the risk of cancer. Vitamin C is also known to inhibit the spread of cancer in the body by neutralizing certain enzymes produced by the cancer cells that lead to metastasis. Minerals, on the other hand, are the building blocks of life. They allow our bodies to digest food, absorb nutrients and keep the alkaline pH balance. While an overdose of multivitamins and minerals is not advisable, regular intake, as prescribed by the oncologist, contributes significantly in the war against cancer.

We are what we eat. What we think. And what we are is collectively controlled by the mind-body continuum. Governed by laws that do not differ from one individual to the other. The same laws of the mind-body continuum exist now as they did over a thousand years ago. However, when any part of our body gets riddled with cancer, it follows its own rules. It's own regulations. Each cancer is unique. Each has its own set of haphazard rules and regulations unmindful of the other. Its own peculiar behaviour. At one instant of time the tiny, individual cell behaves with dignity. The next moment, when influenced by a malignant cell, it starts behaving haphazardly. Joining the group that already exists. Adding to the cancer colony. Expanding the internal destruction and deterioration that, more often than not, will take its own time to get detected. It's own time to get healed.

If, however, we have to protect our various parts of the body from such havoc created by a group of cells, we have to build a strong immune system that can ward off the cancer attack, right in its very infancy. A number of oncologists acknowledge that cancer can be treated by strengthening the patient's own immune system to fight off the disease. Cancer can be considered an immune system deficiency disease, a disease in which the immune system has been compromised. As a cancer patient, it is essential to 'shift' the balance of the diet away from a high fat content diet to one that is protein-rich and contains more fruits, vegetables and grain foods. Even though food and nutrition are the best remedy, the exact relationship between dietary ingredients and cancer is still elusive.

An alert mind and an alert body are absolutely essential for a strong immune system. All the muscles of the body should be toned up. A daily exercise routine that builds the reserves. Studies have indicated that cancer is more likely to occur in the affluent and the indolent, rather than in the poor and overworked. Higher stress could be a factor. Lack of exercise in the upper socio-economic groups is certainly a critical factor. Also it has been noticed that death rates from cancer are higher among those having occupations involving the least muscular effort.

Once the body is healthy, the mind will automatically get pulled in the same direction. Or the other way round. We should ensure that the mind is forever fertile. Always alert. Trained in the art of diagnosing any misbehavior within its scheme of things. Disallowing any bending of rules. And making sure that the body is not lagging far behind. Better still, the mind-body continuum should be maintained at all times. But this is not to say that people whose mind-body continuum is alert at all times are not prone to cancer. Even those who have kept themselves fighting fit through regular exercise, enjoyed all the benefits of healthy living, they too are susceptible to cancer. But more as exceptions than the rule.

Cancer is not the result of bacteria, a virus or an infection that we get exposed to. And most types of cancer are not hereditary either. The cause of any form of cancer is extremely complex and difficult to pinpoint. Regular exercise, balanced diet and nutrition and healthy living are just a few means of keeping cancer at bay. Of course there are no guarantees. I have understood my cancer as my karma. I have believed all along that my life would have been incomplete without it. By that logic, even if I had indulged in a regular exercise routine, lived a healthy life all my life, my karma that is responsible for my cancer would have ensured that I became a cancer patient at the age of 50 years.

The relationship between exercise and reduced risk of cancer can be the result of the fact that stress in the mind and body can be lowered by exercise. Any form of exercise stimulates the immune system and therefore the natural defenses of the mind and body to fight cancer. Take deep breaths during your morning walks. It is also advisable to sit somewhere and rest for about 10 minutes, blanking out your mind so that you are in a better frame of mind to face the day ahead. Those who exercise frequently are more alert and flexible mentally. They are more self-sufficient and accepting; and are able to cope with stress better. Reduced stress and depression enhances the functioning of the immune system. Thereby the power of the mind-body continuum to ward off malignancy. Daily exercise so as to be fit and alert at all moments not only combats stress and depression but also helps in the entire healing process.

If you have to undergo surgery in any form, exercise should begin after your surgery is over, even when you are weak and still recovering from its after-effects. Your physiotherapist will ensure this. Exercise acts as a catalyst to the healing process. In my case, after my not-so-successful surgery, my physiotherapist taught me the art of breathing the day I was shifted back to my room. Deep breathing exercises, holding of the breath, expanding my lungs and chest, followed by slow release. The same to be repeated 5-10 times each time and about 5-10 times each day. The frequency being increased as time elapsed. In the beginning, even this simple breathing exercise seemed extremely difficult. It was then that I realized that I had never paid any attention all my life to the very basics of my existence. My breathing suddenly became a talked-about subject. Amrita, Malika and Kaveri ensured that I did not ignore the physiotherapist's instructions. As the internal healing process began to take shape, new breathing exercises were introduced. New gadgets to help my breathing and to bring my lungs back to their original shape. And in no time, or so I remember now, the after-effects of the surgery were all behind me.

During the period that I attempted to exercise, I felt the quality of my life improve. A fixed time period every morning was devoted to my walks. Consistency was as important as regularity. Exercise also helped me stay in touch with the outside world. With nature as I walked as briskly as I could in the park. Moving my feet. Swinging my arms as far as possible. Exercising my neck, my shoulders as I walked. Becoming more aware of each part of my body. The morning walks also gave me additional time with myself, since I insisted on walking alone. And the days when the side effects of the chemotherapy were too overpowering, I used mental imagery to ensure that my exercise routine was not skipped. Initially I was very enthusiastic about my exercise, my walks in the park. But as time elapsed and the weather became hot, I became lazy and succumbed to my mental imagery instead of the actual walks. Today, I am not as regular as I used to be. I am able to walk about half the distance every week as compared to what I had originally started with and what my oncologist had advised me at the beginning. I realize that this is not sufficient. And that I must return to my earlier routine as soon as possible.

A word of caution. In the days that you feel better and the side effects of the treatment are minimal, you might be tempted to over exercise. Do not ever forget that the drugs that are being used are the strongest known to mankind. In such a condition, anything that exceeds its limits is not advisable. As a cancer patient, or even otherwise, exercise is your response to the needs of the mind-body continuum. Do not strain yourself. Avoid unnecessary tiring. It could lead to complications.

My experience with cancer thus far has shown me the dire importance of healthy living. This is a judicious combination of proper food and regular physical exercise. This has helped not only in building up my energy and internal strength, but also kept my mind-body active, even in the most adverse situations. Healthy living has made significant contributions to the war effort. My progress in the war, according to the last series of tests, has been encouraging. All of us are eagerly waiting the final outcome. The final assault is at hand. The long ordeal will soon be over hopefully. In my mind, in my body I feel that I have won.

DO'S AND DON'T'S FOR FAMILY AND FRIENDS

DO ENCOURAGE A CANCER PATIENT TO TALK ABOUT HIS CONDITION.
It's a healthy sign if he wants to talk. Don't shut him up or change the subject, thinking you're doing him good by not allowing him to indulge in morbidity. It's not morbid to *him*. It's what he's actually having to live through. The subject isn't taboo. Don't enter his room thinking you must talk about everything except the one thing that's staring you in the face. He needs you to know how he's feeling. Shying away from his experiences will make him feel lonely.

DO HELP HIM TO BE INDEPENDENT.
There is a tendency for people to rush in and support a patient in his moments of weakness, thereby denying him the opportunity of taking care of himself. This kind of support only reinforces the illness. Each attempt he makes to help himself should be encouraged as a sign of his own inner strength. Help him to help himself. Support his independence rather than his weakness. If you reserve your attention and love for the times when he is weak, his own initiative to improve will weaken.

DO PRESERVE HIS ROLE WITHIN THE FAMILY UNIT.
By doing so you will ward off potential feelings of helplessness and abandonment. If you've always consulted him on family matters, don't stop. He might be a physical invalid, not a mental one. Normal living patterns within the family unit are extremely important for his self-esteem. Don't cut him off, assuming that he won't be able to cope. Besides, it will make it all the more difficult for him during the rehabilitation period to resume a more functional role.

DO BE AWARE THAT HE WILL SUFFER FROM MOOD SWINGS.
Fear, anger, self-pity, remorse, joy – a cancer patient can experience a gamut of emotions, all in a matter of minutes. The emotional ups and downs can be frightening. Some of these are caused by chemical changes in the body as a result of the treatment. Some, simply because the idea of cancer is hard to bear. Don't molly coddle him, don't present yourself as a willing punching bag, but don't be too harsh on him either. Perhaps you can survive the storms by telling yourself 'this too shall pass'.

DO ASK THE FAMILY IF THEY REQUIRE FINANCIAL HELP.
It is not your duty or responsibility to help but if you're close enough, if you're in a position to do so and want to do so, don't hesitate to ask. Don't hold back thinking that someone's pride might be hurt. Don't imagine there's a phantom bank account somewhere and that you need not enter the picture. Cancer treatment is phenomenally expensive. Unless the family is fabulously wealthy, they're probably devastated financially. The bills are staggering. A friend of my wife's quietly parked her car and chauffeur for three months outside our gate without asking. My wife is one of the proudest women

I know but she accepted the favour gracefully because she was exhausted with the innumerable trips to the hospital.

DO ENQUIRE ABOUT THE WELFARE OF THE FAMILY.
Sometimes it doesn't dawn on people that the family is shattered too. They assume the family has no existence beyond being caretakers of the sick member. The question is always 'How is *he* doing?' But *he* is often doing better than them with all the special food, the care and attention he's getting. The family members often go through deep spells of loneliness. They could also be completely bogged down by bills and chores and hospital duty. Give them a break. Give them time off. Offer to run errands, do the shopping, bring in a meal. Take the kids to a film.

DO ACKNOWLEDGE THAT RELATIONSHIPS WILL CHANGE TEMPORARILY.
This is inevitable for a period. The patient and his family are probably running from one emergency to the next. Their focus changes. They may not respond to old things in the old manner. A friend of mine who used to constantly complain to me about his job carried on doing so after I became a cancer patient. It was like complaining about having no shoes to a man who had no feet. He was fully aware that I had lost my job and moreover, that I was deeply distressed about it. This does not mean you have to constantly watch what you say. Be natural, but be a little sensitive. A strong relationship will survive these temporary changes.

DON'T HIDE WHEN YOU FIRST HEAR THE NEWS.
It's human to want to do so but deeply hurtful for the patient and his family. They'd like to hide too, from the reality of what has hit them, but they can't. If you care, take the plunge. Pick up that phone or ring that doorbell. Tell them you're shocked, tell them you can't bear what you've just heard, say *anything,* howsoever inadequate or clumsy but don't hide. Being cowardly in the face of someone else's misfortune can permanently affect a relationship. Some people I know turned paralyzed on me when they heard I had cancer. When they finally summoned up the courage to face me it was too late. The sad part was that I knew they cared.

DON'T OVERSTAY WHEN YOU VISIT.
Make no mistake, it's a traumatized home you're visiting. Cancer isn't the flu. Don't casually stay on for dinner, for instance, like you might have in the old days. The patient longs to see you but he might be low on energy – physical, emotional, financial. One particular couple did this to me repeatedly. They did it out of love but sheer exhaustion made me avoid them eventually. It's sad and ironical when a cancer patient starts avoiding someone because you would imagine he would want to hang on to every friend he can get. Both sides end up the losers.

DON'T SMOKE IN HIS PRESENCE.
Smokers are usually terrified in the presence of a cancer patient. They have no idea whether a few puffs are acceptable or not. No, they are not, but at the same time there is no need to feel stricken if you must smoke. A cancer patient will not collapse, or get enraged, or feel hurt if you take out a cigarette. Just don't light up in front of him. Use the garden. It's positively harmful for him. That it's harmful for *you* is your

business. Conversely, cancer patients themselves should be sensitive enough to avoid large parties where smoking is inevitable. I once found myself alone in a drawing room on a cold winter's day with the rest of the party shivering on the porch!

DON'T BE NEGATIVE IN HIS PRESENCE.

If you're by nature a grumbler or a whiner you can't suddenly change your personality but do try and curb your negativity in his presence. He is probably fighting his own depression. A cheerful demeanor will not indicate that you do not care. My sister-in-law Shiela used to *enter* my room singing. I am not suggesting everyone do so but her sheer presence banished the sense of doom from my home. A positive atmosphere helps greatly in recovery.

DON'T TREAT HIM LIKE A MORON.

He's lost control of his body and his life already and needs to hang on to his self-esteem. Help him to help himself as much as possible. If he refuses to eat don't speak to him like he were an errant child. If he's undergoing treatment he's genuinely nauseous. But if he behaves unreasonable, tick him off. Don't take self-indulgence or any nonsense from him. He needs assurance that he is still functional as a human being. It's important for him to participate in the normal dynamics of human relationships.

DON'T SHOWER HIM WITH AFFECTION OR PITY.

He is fully aware of the gravity of his situation and your constant kindness can make him nervous. It can make him wonder whether he's dying, whether there's something about his condition you're not telling him.

DON'T ABANDON HIM AS SOON AS HE'S ON HIS FEET. The period of rehabilitation is almost as traumatizing as the illness itself. He is desperately in need of your support just then. Hold his hand a while longer, even if you're exhausted by then. Cancer patients find it difficult to slip back into society immediately. He could be emotionally drained. He might have lost his confidence.

MYTHS AND MISCONCEPTIONS ABOUT CANCER

MYTH: CANCER IS CONTAGIOUS.
REALITY: Cancer is the result of chromosome damage, and is therefore not communicable. One cannot 'catch' cancer by touching, hugging or being near a patient. At one time, when little was known about its cause, people would shy away from a cancer patient for fear of bringing the disease upon themselves. There's no need to avoid someone who has cancer. You can't catch it. It is, on the other hand, possible to catch diseases and viruses that can lead to it. Around 15% of cancers worldwide are caused this way. Cervical cancer, for example, is virtually always (99.7%) a consequence of HPV, a sexually transmitted infection. Liver cancer is 100 times more likely in hepatitis B victims, which is why it's one of the few cancers with a high prevalence in the Third World as compared to the western world.

MYTH: CANCER IS A DISEASE OF OLDER PEOPLE.
REALITY: Cancer can occur at any age. That's why it is so important to have regular medical check-ups and learn all about self-examination. In many cases, the sooner cancer is diagnosed and treated, the better a person's chance for a full recovery. About 40% of all cancer cases occur in those under

the age of 65. Some cancers, such as Hodgkin's and testicular cancer, target the young. This is why it is important to be aware of physical changes, symptoms and lumps at all ages.

MYTH: ALL CANCERS ARE INHERITED.
REALITY: While it is true that having a mother, father, sister or brother, with cancer increases your own risk, it does not automatically guarantee it. Certain cancers do prevail in some families, for example, breast or colon cancers. While the family history of the disease can play a role in developing cancer, it is not a reliable indication. Smoking, alcohol intake, dietary habits, and environmental exposures also increase a person's risk of developing cancer. Many people with one or more risk factors never develop cancer, while others with this disease have no known risk factors.

MYTH: INJURIES CAN CAUSE CANCER.
REALITY: Cuts, bruises, broken bones, etc., do not cause cancer. For instance, bruises or hits to the breast will not cause breast cancer, nor will broken bones cause bone cancer. Injuries may bring a heightened awareness of those areas, making one more conscious of any future symptoms.

MYTH: STRESS CAUSES CANCER.
REALITY: Although stress has been suspected as a risk factor in addictions, obesity, high blood pressure, peptic ulcer, colitis, asthma, insomnia, migraine headaches, lower back pain, physiological disorders and a weakened immunity system, a direct connection to the development of cancer has not yet been proven.

MYTH: CANCER CAUSES PAIN.
REALITY: Some cancers do not cause pain. And more than half of all cancer patients describe their pain as moderate.

The myth of uncontrollable pain is one of the reasons people still fear the disease. Cancer pain can be controlled so that the patient is comfortable. Advanced cancer can certainly cause pain, but in the past 5 to 10 years doctors have become more aware of the need to control this pain and have access to better medication to counter it. Although the pain can't always be eliminated, it may be controlled to the point where it has little to no impact on day-to-day living. The pain associated with cancer is due to a number of reasons. For example, the tumor may be pressing a nerve, interfering with the function of an organ, or it may have invaded a bone and caused a weakening or fracture of the bone. Infection from treatments such as surgery, radiation, or medications may cause pain as well.

MYTH: CANCER PAIN IS UNTREATABLE.
REALITY: For those who do have painful episodes, several treatment options are available. These include pain-relieving drugs, radiation therapy (to shrink a tumor that's causing pain) or surgery (to block nerve pathways that carry pain impulses to your brain).

MYTH: EXTREMELY OVERWEIGHT PEOPLE ARE MORE LIKELY TO DEVELOP CANCER.
REALITY: Some say there is a connection between obesity and cancer but the link is not clear. There are two exceptions, though. Obese women are three to five times more likely to get endometrial (lining of the uterus) cancer and obese post-menopausal women run an increased risk of breast cancer.

MYTH: CANCER MEANS CERTAIN DEATH.
REALITY: Modern medication ensures that most forms of cancer can be treated and controlled. Millions of cancer survivors are living healthy and fruitful lives all over the world.

In America alone, it is estimated that there are approximately seven million people living with a history of cancer. About half of the individuals diagnosed with cancer survive for five years or more, and some forms of cancer are completely treatable if detected early. Even if not entirely treatable, many cases become chronic conditions needing attention, somewhat like diabetes or heart disease, and patients focus on living and coping rather than believing that their situation is hopeless. Early detection is the key to curing cancer. That's why regular screenings and self-examinations are so important. Two-thirds of patients diagnosed with cancer of the breast, tongue, mouth, colon, rectum, cervix or prostate survive five years or more. With early detection, about 95 percent would survive. No one knows exactly how each patient will respond to treatment but more and more people are surviving cancer.

MYTH: ALL CANCERS ARE EQUALLY BAD AND REFLECT THE SAME GRIM OUTLOOK.
REALITY: Cancers of different organs carry a very different prognosis. While some progress rapidly without treatment, others develop at a very slow pace. For example, certain cancers of the skin (basal cell carcinoma), the thyroid and the prostate, proceed at a very slow pace, and may take years before becoming life-threatening.

MYTH: A POSITIVE ATTITUDE IS ALL YOU NEED TO BEAT CANCER.
REALITY: There's no scientific proof that a positive attitude gives you an advantage in cancer treatment or improves your chance of being cured. What a positive attitude can do is improve the quality of your life during cancer treatment. You may be more likely to stay active, maintain ties with family and friends and continue social activities. In turn, this may

enhance your feeling of well-being and help you find the strength to deal with your cancer. A positive attitude may also help you become an active and responsible partner with your doctor during treatment.

MYTH: WE WILL SOON HAVE A CURE FOR CANCER.

REALITY: Despite advances in research we still don't know what causes a cell to become cancerous and why some people with cancer do better than others. Finding the cure for cancer is, in fact, proving to be more complex than mastering the engineering and physics required for space flight.

MYTH: DRUG COMPANIES AND THE FOOD AND DRUG ADMINISTRATION ARE BLOCKING OR WITHHOLDING NEW CANCER TREATMENTS.

REALITY: If you're going through cancer treatment it's natural to feel frustrated and wish there were a magic cure. You might even wonder if a new treatment is being withheld. That's not the case. Your doctor and the FDA, which approves new drugs, are your allies. As such, they make your safety a high priority. Unfortunately, scientific studies to determine a treatment's safety and effectiveness take time. That may create the feeling that new treatments are being blocked. Thorough testing has kept many unsafe and ineffective drugs from being used.

MYTH: REGULAR CHECK-UPS AND TODAY'S MEDICAL TECHNOLOGY CAN DETECT CANCER EARLY.

REALITY: Routine screening has clearly led to a decrease in deaths from several cancers, including cervix, breast and colon cancers. Regular medical care can indeed increase your ability to detect cancer early but it can't guarantee it. Cancer is a complicated disease, and there's no sure way to always spot it. Cancer cells can grow anywhere in your body, often deep within it. Until the cancer reaches a certain size, there isn't a technology or an examination capable of detecting it. By the time you can feel a breast cancer lump, for instance, the cancer may have been there four to six years.

MYTH: UNDERGOING CANCER TREATMENT MEANS YOU CAN'T WORK OR LEAD A NORMAL LIFE.
REALITY: Many people do work full or part time during their treatment. A great deal of time and effort has gone into making it easier for people to live a more normal life during and after their treatment. The result is you're often able to stay active during your treatment.

MYTH: CANCER TREATMENT IS WORSE THAN THE DISEASE.
REALITY: Many people fear cancer treatment more than the disease itself, but every year new techniques or devices improve procedures and make the treatment easier to tolerate. New medications also do a better job of controlling or eliminating side effects, and reconstructive surgery can sometimes minimize physical changes caused by surgery.

MYTH: ALL CANCERS GET TREATED THE SAME WAY.
REALITY: Different types of cancer vary in their rates of growth, patterns of spread, and responses to different types of treatment. That's why people with cancer need treatment that is aimed at their specific form of the disease.

MYTH: CANCER CAN'T BE PREVENTED.
REALITY: The sense that cancer can strike anyone, anywhere, any time is part of what makes it so frightening. While it's true that many cancers aren't preventable, many are. 90% of skin cancers could be prevented if people protected themselves from the sun's rays. In addition, all cancers

caused by tobacco use and heavy drinking are preventable. Overall, researchers estimate that if people applied everything known about cancer prevention to their lives, up to two-thirds of cancers wouldn't occur. Modern medicine has learned a lot about cancer. The most common risks which we have become aware of in recent years are smoking, exposure to asbestos, overexposure to the sun, ionizing radiation, certain viral infections such as HIV and hepatitis, and exposure to a variety of chemicals such as phosphorus, silica, etc. We have also learned that various types of diet can reduce the risk of cancer, for example eating non-fatty foods reduces the risk of cancer of the intestines. Also, simple self-examinations, awareness of any unusual changes in our body or body functions and regular medical screenings to achieve early detection of more common types of cancer can make a crucial difference in our survival and quality of life.

MYTH: EVERYONE WITH THE SAME KIND OF CANCER GETS THE SAME TREATMENT.
REALITY: Your doctor tailors your treatment for you. What treatment you receive depends on where your cancer is, how much it has spread and how it's affecting your body functions and your general health. In addition, cells from the same type of cancer may have different features. These differences can affect how the cells respond to treatment, which in turn may influence your doctor's recommendations.

MYTH: GOOD PEOPLE DON'T GET CANCER.
REALITY: In ancient times, illness was viewed as punishment for bad actions or thoughts. In some cultures that view is still held. If this were true, though, how would we explain the 6-month-old or the newborn who gets cancer? There is absolutely no evidence that you get cancer because you

deserve it.

MYTH: HAVING A TUMOR MEANS YOU HAVE CANCER.
REALITY: It is important to realize that not all tumors are cancerous. Benign or non-cancerous tumors do not spread and, with very rare exceptions, are not life-threatening.

MYTH: URBAN LIFE GIVES YOU CANCER.
REALITY: No, there is no difference in incidence rate between the town and the countryside. The same doesn't seem to be true, though, for survival rates. Studies around the world indicate that in rural areas, patients with stomach cancer were four times more likely to die before the cancer was diagnosed. For breast cancer, it is three times. This is only because country dwellers have less access to specialist care.

MYTH: MOST CANCER TREATMENTS ARE INEFFECTIVE OR MINIMALLY EFFECTIVE.
REALITY: While it is true that the success of cancer therapy depends on the type of cancer, its site of origin, its time of detection, the degree of cancer differentiation and its rate of growth, in many cases, treatment is curative or prolongs life with a good quality of life for many years. Today, physicians have a great variety of treatments for cancer ranging from surgery to special techniques of radiation, powerful chemotherapy and hormonal treatments.

MYTH: RADIATION THERAPY MAKES ONE RADIOACTIVE.
REALITY: Radiation therapy will not make the patient radioactive. The body does not act like a battery, storing and emitting the radiation. When the linear accelerator is shut off, the radiation ceases. There is no need to restrain from having contact, such as hugging, kissing, touching or sexual relations, with someone receiving treatment. However, patients who

have received prostate seed implants are advised not to have small children sit on their laps, or come into contact with pregnant women during the first couple of months following their procedure.

MYTH: ALL TREATMENTS HAVE THE SAME SIDE EFFECTS, SUCH AS HAIR LOSS, NAUSEA AND VOMITING.
REALITY: The type of treatment and area being treated will determine the side effects. For instance, radiation patients will lose hair only in the area being treated. Also, not everyone will experience the same side effects to the same degree. The side effects also depend on the treatment and the drugs used. Besides, medication is available to prevent and combat most side effects of the treatment.

MYTH: RADIATION TREATMENT IS PAINFUL.
REALITY: As with an x-ray, one will not feel the radiation being administered. Also, today's technology enables the radiation oncologist to minimize damage to healthy tissue by focusing the treatment to the tumor area.

MYTH: CHEMOTHERAPY IS ONE DRUG.
REALITY: Chemotherapy involves a wide range of chemicals, dosages and combinations. Different combinations may be used for specific cancers.

MYTH: SURGERY CAUSES CANCER TO SPREAD BY EXPOSING IT TO AIR.
REALITY: Exposure to air does not cause cancer spread. Surgery is used to remove cancerous cells from the body. During surgery, it may be determined that the cancer has spread to the lymph nodes, requiring their removal as well. Sometimes, additional surgery is performed to remove cancer that has already spread to other parts of the body, or

to remove cancer that has reoccurred at the original site. All of these may lend to the myth of surgery causing the spread of cancer. Also, you may feel worse during your recovery than you did before surgery, making you believe your surgery caused your cancer to spread. 'Air hitting the tumor' does not cause cancer to spread, although removing the main tumor mass may facilitate the growth of cancer that has spread (metastasis). Although it's possible that during surgery your doctor may find the cancer more widespread than previously thought, an operation can't cause cancer to spread nor can it cause cancer to start. Surgically removing cancer cells is often the first and most important treatment.

MYTH: MAN-MADE CHEMICALS ARE TO BLAME FOR INCREASING CANCER INCIDENCE.
REALITY: Not really. Estimates indicate that 1% of cancers are caused by food additives and another about 1% a result of man-made chemicals. However, a 1999 German report and a more recent one by the US Environmental Protection Agency estimated that about 12% of cancers in industrialized countries were the result of dioxins. Other scientists, while not disputing that dioxins are poisonous, doubt that they are ingested in sufficient quantities and point out that there is no causal link evidence.

MYTH: EVERY SECOND PERSON SEEMS TO BE A CANCER PATIENT.
REALITY: In the US, 48% of men and 37% of women will get cancer at some point during their life. The UK figure is a little lower. According to the Imperial Cancer Research Fund, just over one in three will get cancer and one in four will die of it. Currently, the male five-year survival rate is just 31%, while the female is 43%. Five years is the cancer experts' preferred

definition of 'survival'.

MYTH: VEGETARIANS DON'T GET CANCER AS OFTEN AS NON-VEGETARIANS.

REALITY: Fruit and vegetables cannot keep cancer away. Experts have pointed out, however, that red meat and saturated fats are laden with chemicals that lead to cancer. Fruits and vegetables, on the other hand, contain phytochemicals and antioxidants that fight cancer. The conclusion therefore was that meat-eating leads to cancer. A recent research indicates that vegetarians are just as likely to die of bowel cancer as meat eaters. Nor was there any difference in breast, prostate, lung or stomach cancer. Another study, by the US National Cancer Institute, found that people on a low-fat diet seemed to stand as much chance of developing pre-cancerous growths in their colons as those who ate meat regularly.

MYTH: ONLY WOMEN GET BREAST CANCER.

REALITY: Men can also get breast cancer, although it is rare. If you notice a lump that does not go away in your breast tissue, make sure you see a doctor.

MYTH: IF YOU HAVE A PAINFUL LUMP IN YOUR BREAST, IT MUST BE CANCER.

REALITY: Most likely not. 90% of breast cancer tumors are not painful. It is far more likely to be an abscess, which is always painful.

MYTH: ONLY WOMEN WHO ARE OVER FIFTY GET BREAST CANCER.

REALITY: While it is true that the disease is found in 78% of women in this age group, there is a significant number of cases found in women under the age of 30. In fact, it is found at a more advanced stage in younger women. This may be the result of delay in diagnosis because they have not been part of a regular screening process such as a breast self-examination.

MYTH: SMALL BREASTED WOMEN DO NOT GET BREAST CANCER.

REALITY: Every woman is at risk regardless of breast size, race or socio-economic status. One in every eight women will get breast cancer and 40% of this group will die from it within ten years.

MYTH: MORE MEN DIE OF PROSTATE CANCER THAN WOMEN OF BREAST CANCER.

REALITY: Breast cancer is the leading killer disease for women between 35 and 54. According to some statistics, the lifetime risk is one in eight. Prostate cancer, by contrast, is a one in 14 shot, with a 41% survival rate. Breast cancer survival rates are rapidly improving, though.

MYTH: REGULAR YEARLY BREAST EXAMINATIONS DETECT ALL BREAST CANCER IN ITS EARLY STAGES.

REALITY: While breast cancers may be found earlier with regular examinations, it is wrong to believe that all cancers will be detected. Most breast cancers have been present for 8-10 years before a lump is found. Even mammograms are not 100% accurate and up to 40% of mammograms do not detect breast cancer in younger women.

MYTH: ONLY WOMEN WITH A FAMILY HISTORY GET BREAST CANCER.

REALITY: The majority of women who get breast cancer have no family history and have none of the identifiable risk factors. However, if there is a family history, the chances of breast cancer are increased and tests should be done at an earlier age and with a higher frequency. Tests can also be done for the BRAC1, BRAC2 and P53 genes and changes (mutations) in these genes if they have been inherited. These genes are responsible for over 90% of inherited cancer, and if these genes have been inherited, chances of getting the disease by the age of 60 increase to 85-90%. If these genes are not inherited, the risk is only slightly higher than for all women.

MYTH: BREAST CANCER IS KILLING MORE AND MORE YOUNG WOMEN.

REALITY: Death rates have been reduced by 30% in young and middle-aged victims, mostly because of the efficacy of Tamoxifen, a cheap and effective drug which blocks hormone receptors on cancer cells, interfering with their growth. It probably saves more lives than any other form of non-surgical cancer treatment. In younger women, chemotherapy after surgery has made a big difference to death rates.

MYTH: VIRGINS ARE MORE LIKELY TO BE BREAST CANCER PATIENTS.

REALITY: Virgins are more likely to get it because they don't have children. Breast cancer is closely linked to oestrogen levels. Having babies, particularly when you're young, lowers the risk. By contrast, the fewer children you have, the greater your risk. Other risks are late menopause and having a first child after 30 years of age. The older you are, the greater the danger.

MYTH: CERVICAL CANCER CAN BE A RESULT OF PROMISCUITY.

REALITY: The younger a woman is when she first has sex and the more sexual partners she has in her lifetime, the greater her chance of getting cervical cancer. That's because it's one of the few cancers caused by something you can catch. More than 99% of women who get it have the Human Papilloma Virus (HPV). Male promiscuity is also a major cause. Women who have had only one partner also get HPV. Male promiscuity, combined with lower hygiene levels, is often the problem in the Third World. Men catch HPV from prostitutes and infect their wives and lovers.

MYTH: MALE CIRCUMCISION LEADS TO PREVENTION OF CERVICAL CANCER.
REALITY: There is some evidence for this. In India, Muslim women have a lower rate of cervical cancer than Hindus and Christians. It certainly seems to prevent penile cancer, which is virtually never seen in circumcised men.

MYTH: FLYING GIVES YOU LEUKEMIA.
REALITY: As a long-term commercial pilot, you are five times more likely to get leukemia. The effect is related to the high number of hours flown and only applies to those who have put in more than 5,000 hours. It is a purely professional risk and most likely caused by cosmic radiation that increases with altitude. So the higher you fly, the more marked the effect and presumably Concorde pilots run the greatest risk.

MYTH: EVERY MAN, IF HE LIVES LONG ENOUGH, WILL EVENTUALLY GET PROSTATE CANCER.
REALITY: Probably. The death toll has doubled over the last 20 years. 40% of all 80-year-old men have prostate cancer and this was established through post-mortems. Many won't know they've got it, as it develops slowly and they'll die of something else first. The incidence increases with age. So if men lived to over 120 or so, it is possible they would all get prostate cancer. But not necessarily die of it. It looks as if there could well be a form of prostate cancer that just sits there and grows very slowly.

LIFE AFTER CANCER

I still remember the day when the last of the series of tests confirmed that there was no sign of malignancy in my lungs. On the x-rays and CT scans the patch appeared like a scar, a tell-tale sign that at some stage in the past there had been something wrong with my lungs. I realized that I would have to live with this abnormality, the same way as I would have to live with the scar of my surgery. But the fact was that I was in remission.

That was about three months ago. Today there was another major victory. Today I was able to brush my hair for the first time in about eight months. The loss of hair as a result of chemotherapy was for me the biggest setback that I had to cope with during my treatment. I had always been extremely proud of my hair. As I ran my brush through my hair for the first time and felt my hair responding, I was overjoyed. In the last few weeks, Amrita and my daughters had often seen me standing in front of the mirror. Trying to brush my hair and not succeeding. I know they wondered at my strange and undying love for my hair. They just did not understand my trauma. The loneliness of a man with no hair on his head.

The worst was now behind me. I was in remission. I had

brushed my hair for the first time this morning. And all this was cause for celebration. It was a joyous occasion. Some months back, however, I had decided that celebrations in my life no longer had the same relevance or meaning as earlier. I knew cancer played by its own rules. It obeyed its own haphazard laws. Cancer once experienced meant it could come back. So many patients I had met at hospital were coping with treatment for the second and third and fourth time.

I was confident that, having won my war against cancer, I could overcome anything. Everything. My life was back to normal. Some major changes had occurred. Healthy living was one of them. Absence of tobacco was another. Celebrations did not have the same meaning anymore as they had before the cancer was diagnosed. Everything in life now seemed transient. What are we celebrating when we celebrate? Marriage is one the most important occasions that calls for a celebration. Yet there is an air of gloom as the bride departs, leaving her parents' home forever. Happiness for one can be a sad occasion for another. Everything is relative.

Cancer had changed a number of things in my life. My values. My outlook. My inner being. I was not the same person anymore. The person that I was before my diagnosis. Even the person that I was during my treatment. How had cancer changed so much of me? Or why had I allowed cancer to change me thus? Most life-threatening diseases have a similar effect. A long period of treatment can cause major changes. Not many things annoyed me. Irritated me. During my days of treatment I had become more of a loner than ever before. Very rarely did I step out. And mostly my trips were visits to the hospital. I began to realize the enormity of what I had been through last year. My close shave with possible death. The 'why *me*?' that had been bottled up deep, deep inside surfaced once more. I had started to question my cancer. Why had my life been so adversely affected? What had I done to deserve this? I felt remorse. I felt anger. I felt one year of my life had been wasted. I felt cheated. Why was all this so important now? Especially since I was in remission. I could not find the answers and decided to see a therapist. She clarified my new feelings towards the cancer. She informed me that sooner or later all this had to surface. Very few, she said, could survive something like cancer without feelings of anger. Feelings of remorse could surface much after the treatment was over. I just had to accept them the same way as I had accepted my cancer. I just had to move forward in my life accepting all that had happened. I had to stop living in the past.

The tell-tale signs of cancer were still very obvious. Though hidden for most of the day, they became clearly visible when I bathed every morning. The chemo-port was still there. The slight swelling just below my left shoulder was a reminder of its presence. Also, it had to be flushed every month with Heplock injections so as to ensure that its internal tubes were not blocked. I still had to meet my oncologist every month for regular check-ups. And every second or third month, undergo a chest x-ray. And a CT scan. Blood tests. Ultrasound imaging. The scar from the surgery had disfigured me for life. Most of the time this did not bother me. Except when I saw myself in the mirror. When I felt the scar with my hands. The other damage resulting from the side effects of the drugs, including my impaired hearing and the variable blood pressure had returned to normal. Even the hair on my body was coming back. It was thick. It was black. It was good to be whole again. I could walk down the road holding my head high. I felt proud of my victory. The long, arduous days of the war that I had fought had not gone in vain. I was set to take on the whole world.

Before I did I had to ensure that the chances of recurrence of the cancer were minimized. My oncologist had prescribed a course of multivitamins and antioxidants. I went back to my ayurved, who prescribed a series of medicines that he said would prevent the return of cancer. Build my immunity. Soon I noticed that my feet were swelling. During the next monthly check-up, my oncologist said it was a problem of water retention. I was advised to have my ayurvedic medication analyzed at a laboratory. This was when I discovered that the medicine was nothing but steroids. Naturally, it had to be stopped immediately. I was shattered. I had no other option available to me to prevent the recurrence of cancer. I consulted the experts I knew in alternative medicine. I switched to homeopathy. While I knew that there were no rules that were applicable to cancer, the homeopathic treatment made me feel somewhat safe. As did the antioxidants and the multivitamins. Even after remission, I was considered a high-risk patient. Chances of recurrence were high. It was precisely for this reason that I still walked around with my chemo-port. If maintained well, the life of the chemo-port was about two years. I was advised not to have it removed just in case chemotherapy had to be administered again.

Living with the fear of recurrence is frightening. I had discussed my case history through e-mail with oncologists at a cancer hospital in Houston, Texas. And their reply was the same. Although in remission, I had no cause to celebrate. Did I have the mental energy and the inner strength to fight another war? Would the formula work again if required? Or would I have to develop a new battle plan? Did I have it in me to go through all that I had gone though all over again if necessary? Equally important was the consideration that I could not let my family and friends go through the trauma again. I just had to extend my period of remission. I just had to ensure that there was no chance of recurrence of cancer. I had to follow a definite plan. A strategy. Healthy living. Chanting and meditation. Minimum of stress and tension. On my part I was taking all the precautions that were possible. Changes in health were the result of changes in the balance of the mind-body continuum. The mind had to be alert at all times to accept the needs of the body. And the body too had to be always in tune with the mind. Any slight deviation, however insignificant or small would upset the balance. I had tried all this last year during the days I was fighting the war. I was convinced something new, something different, was also required.

Exercise had been one of my failures in all my efforts in healthy living since last year. I had let my oncologist down on this score. I had let myself down. Any form of exercise had always been difficult for me. Ever since my treatment was over, I had been putting on weight. Regular exercise was now even more critical. I restarted my yoga classes. The yoga instructor came home three times a week. Yoga also helped me tone up the mind-body continuum. I felt more relaxed than ever before. My inner resolve was strengthened further. I found new ways to stay alert. And fit. Life after cancer also meant doing things that I had never done before. Completing all the tasks at hand since my life span had been shortened somewhat.

Discussions about death are always morbid. Irrespective of age and health status, the most difficult and fearsome fact of life is death. As cancer patients we are always close to death. The failure to acknowledge the possibility of death gives rise to all the fears. The destruction and devastation that cancer causes is like a lingering death that is an emotional, psychological and financial drain on the patient. On the family and friends. As a cancer patient it is important to confront the possibility of death openly and be somewhat ready for it. It can strike any time. Even when you are in good health. Crossing a road and being hit by a moving vehicle. While driving, a sudden loss of concentration. And so on. Sometimes the death of someone close to you can help you come to terms with your own feelings about death.

Once you are diagnosed as a cancer patient, during your treatment, or even when you are in remission, you live with a feeling of resignation. A realization that you may be living on borrowed time. Facing death does not diminish hope even though your hopes and desires may undergo a total sea change. Even a dying person still hopes for a cure. Or death with dignity. Death without pain or fear. Not every cancer patient experiences physical pain towards the last stages. Pain can result from a tumor pushing on a nerve, a vital organ or other parts of the body. And in most cases oncologists can offer palliative treatment to relieve the pain. It is important to know that most of the myths and misconceptions patients have about pain have no basis.

Managing physical pain is the simpler part of life after cancer. Emotional pain and fear are far worse. I had never been unemployed for so long. It was nearly 10 months. Though I had been for a few job interviews, nothing had materialized. Every day I had sent my papers to various corporate houses. In response to advertisements in the newspapers. To friends. Yet there was no job in sight. It remained a distant dream. As time went by I became more and more depressed. I began to feel unwanted. Was this why I had fought so hard against cancer? In the beginning, the corporate world appeared strange. Even when I visited offices that I was familiar with. Cancer had gnawed at my confidence levels. I felt shattered. My knees felt weak the first time I entered an office. I wanted to go back home. I thought I would collapse. I would faint. As days passed, I became more confident. But the emotional stress of being unemployed continued to increase. Chanting helped. So did meditation. But each time I set out of the house for an interview or a meeting, the tension was obvious. It was written all over my face. Maybe this was the reason a job was alluding me. We were sinking deeper and deeper into debt. And then one fine morning everything fell into place. I found a job. The same day my father passed away.

If you are being interviewed for a job, do not disclose your cancer history unless it is relevant. Prospective employers are not entitled to know everything about your medical history. You should only volunteer information that directly applies to your ability to perform the job functions. And if your cancer is not relevant, which in most cases it won't be, you are under no obligation to bring it up. However, always be truthful if someone asks about your health status and more so, once you are offered the job. In the beginning of my hunt for a job, I overdid the honesty bit. Or maybe my baldness had made my cancer history obvious. But I was proud of being a cancer survivor. Besides, a lot of people already knew about my situation. When I found that being totally honest was not getting me anywhere, was not getting me my job, I decided to keep quiet about the cancer.

Now about a year has passed since my cancer was first diagnosed. Its nearly five months since I was labeled a cancer survivor. And one month since I started working again. The only way to cope with life after cancer is to integrate the experiences of cancer with your daily life. This is easier said than done. Not so long ago you had seen it as your worst enemy. How is it possible then to coexist with it now? The truth is, you have no other option. There is no way you can pretend you have not been a cancer patient. No way that your friends, and those who know about your medical history, will not label you a cancer survivor. Life after cancer has to be lived with a new form of courage, hope, joy, compassion and faith. It must have a new meaning. New challenges. The memories of cancer can, and may, fade with time. Or they may continue to haunt you forever. Here again, the choice is yours.

How each cancer survivor copes with life after cancer is different. How one responds to any situation is conditioned by many factors. And one of them is how you as a patient survived some of the worst moments of your cancer. The lessons that you learned. The inner strength you gained. Your positive attitude. These images get transfixed in your mind-body continuum.

Once you are touched with cancer it becomes a part of you forever. You are either a cancer patient or a cancer survivor. Even if the doctors pronounce you cured, you do not have 100% proof that all the malignant cells in your body have been destroyed. All the cancer has been flushed out. You can never go back to the life you lived before the diagnosis. No matter how much you may want it, and wish it, to happen. Cancer alters your mind-body continuum. You exist in a new balance. Your chemistry changes. New equations govern your life. Your relationships with your family. With your friends. With your work and living environment. As my therapist advised me during one of our many meetings. After coping with cancer, almost every experience that follows appears trivial. This led to a lot of frustration. A lot of despair. Sometimes, I had this feeling that I was superior when I looked at my family, my friends, around me. I was special. I had fought a war and won. They hadn't.

The quiet that follows cancer treatment is sometimes as difficult as what has gone before. You are no longer the centre of attention. No longer does your family treat you with the same consideration as they did when you were undergoing treatment. Or your friends for that matter. They don't come and visit you as often as they did earlier. Or inquire about your health status. You are left coping with the new you. As a survivor only you realize what is happening. Others around you don't. And this strains your relationships. All your relationships. With people. With family. With friends. A relationship is a two-way process. Others around you may have remained the same. You have changed forever. And therefore, all your relationships have to have a new meaning. A different form.

At the hospital I had made friends with fellow cancer patients that I had met. Each had been fighting his or her personal war. A few days back I was informed that one of them was not as lucky as I had been. I attended his funeral. And since then a lot has changed inside me. We are not the ones to choose who survives and who does not. Our life is not at the cost of another. After the funeral, I have felt more like my old self again. I have begun to trust my mind, my body. I am glad I survived. Yet at times I feel guilty. The same kind of guilt that I had felt as a child on days I had lied to my

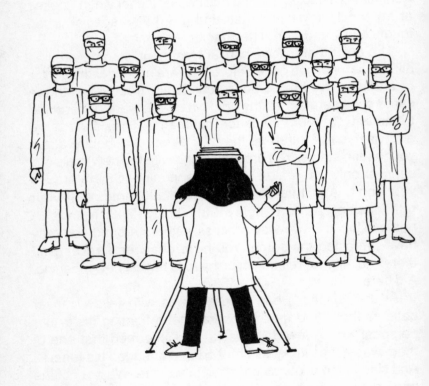

"Say cheese!"

mother. Or before the diagnosis, the time I had told Amrita that I had been hard at work when actually I had gone for a drink with the boys. It felt wonderful to get some of the old feelings back. Even if they arose out of guilt. Did this mean that I was putting my cancer behind me? Time was a great healer. Could time also heal my deep cancer wounds? My pain. My anguish. My missed job opportunity last year, the dream that my cancer had shattered. Since the funeral, my inner strength has increased. I am now able to cope with my emotional and physical needs in a more organized manner. I am quite willing to wage another war, if the cancer ever came back. The feeling of guilt about being a cancer survivor, and its similarity to earlier feelings of guilt, has been the turning point.

Surviving cancer is about living a day at a time. It's about having the best quality of life that is possible. One of my new friends, a breast cancer patient, told me that the only difference between life before and after cancer was that earlier she could plan her future with some amount of certainty. As a cancer survivor her future had shrunk, and it was becoming more and more difficult to plan more than three or four months at a time. There is no way she could plan her life five years ahead, even when she knew she had been in remission for over five years. Cancer is totally unpredictable. Before cancer, most of us live our lives never thinking about cancer. Or even if we do, we think it can never happen to us. Just the knowledge that it can, and has, changes everything.

As cancer survivors, we should reach out and grasp each day as if we had only that day to live. Experience and enjoy every moment of our lives. After all, we only have one life to live. We have our own individual goals. We should rise far above all that we consider trivial in our life, in our environment.

Look back at the memories of our lives without cancer. If we felt the need to do something, we just did it. The same still holds true now as it did earlier. Never let anybody put you down. Or let them discriminate against you because of your cancer. If you have a dream, then act on it.

From this year onwards, I decided I would have two birthdays. June 14, the day I was born. And October 30, the day I won my first war against cancer. From now onwards, I will try harder, work longer, and achieve more. My life will be lived with passion. With zest. With a sense of joy, creativity and spontaneity. Enthusiasm, excitement and fulfillment. Through cancer I have received a new gift of life. The joy of cancer is not about what cancer does to us. To our mind. To our body. It is about how we perceive what has happened to us. And what is happening to us. It's about finding a positive for every negative. A good in every bad. And converting all our setbacks into new challenges to be faced. New wars to be fought and won. We have learned the art of the making the mind and body work together. In perfect harmony. The cancer has developed our mind-body continuum and taken it to another level. A higher plane. A new balance which in many ways is superior to what existed before. We have learned to confront our worst fears.

In 1979, the Indian Cancer Society asked
Ogilvy & Mather to develop a multimedia communication
program to generate greater awareness about cancer,
with a focus on early detection. This exercise of using
mass-media to educate people about cancer was
the first of its kind in India. Before the campaign was
launched, the free cancer check-up clinics in Bombay city
received on an average of about three patients a month
and as result of the awareness that was created,
over 3,000 people a month started availing of this facility.

The print media campaign, which is reproduced
on the following pages, won many national awards and
also received international recognition.

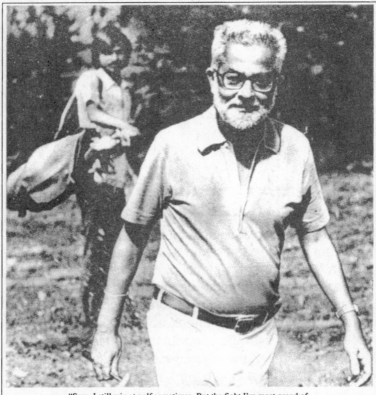

"Sure, I still win at golf sometimes. But the fight I'm most proud of,
is the fight I won against cancer!" *says Prahlad Mehta*

Life after cancer...it's worth living

When Prahlad Mehta first noticed the lump on the side of his neck, it was tiny and painless.

"I wasn't prepared for the doctor's diagnosis," he says. "Cancer of the lymph nodes."

Prahlad was treated at the Tata Memorial Hospital in Bombay-- one of the most modern cancer centres in the world.

He was lucky. His cancer had been detected early and he recovered very fast.

"In fact," says Prahlad, "I never missed a single day's work or a single weekend's golf-- right through the treatment!"

Prahlad is just one of thousands of Indians who are winning their fight against cancer. But it isn't luck that saves them. It is early treatment.

In recent years, we have developed many effective drugs to control cancer.

Today, most cancers are curable, if treated early. That's why a yearly cancer check-up is so necessary for every adult.

We have several free check-up centres all over Bombay. Find out which is the one closest to you.

Phone: 231417 for a free cancer check-up.

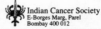

Indian Cancer Society
E-Borges Marg, Parel
Bombay 400 012

O&M/3756

"Sure, I still win at golf sometimes. But the fight I'm most proud of is the fight I won against cancer!" says Prahlad Mehta

When Prahlad Mehta first noticed the lump on the side of his neck, it was tiny and painless.

"I wasn't prepared for the doctor's diagnosis," he says. "Cancer of the lymph nodes."

Prahlad was treated at the Tata Memorial Hospital in Bombay — one of the most modern cancer centres in the world.

He was lucky. His cancer had been detected early and he recovered very fast.

"In fact," says Prahlad, "I never missed a single day's work or a single weekend's golf — right through the treatment."

Prahlad is just one of the thousands of Indians who are winning their fight against cancer. But it isn't luck that saves them. It is early treatment.

In recent years we have developed many effective drugs to control cancer.

Today, most cancers are curable, if treated early. That's why a yearly cancer check-up is so necessary for every adult.

We have several free check-up centres all over Bombay. Find out which is the one closest to you.

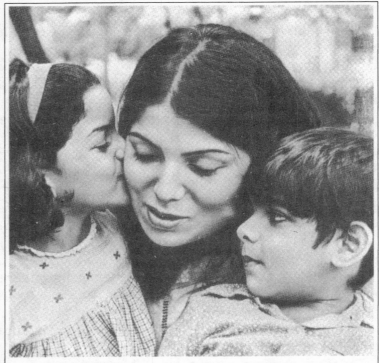

Don't delay your cancer check-up this year.
The lives of others depend on it

Take a little time off today, for the sake of someone you love... and drop in for a cancer check-up. Cancer will strike 5,000 more people in Bombay city alone this year.

The symptoms are so minor at first, you could have cancer and not know it. Yet, our chances of curing cancer are best, when it's detected early. That's why an annual check-up is so important.

Remember...cancer doesn't always happen to someone else. Get a free check-up at any of our centres.

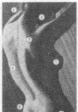

Look for these early warning signals of cancer:
1. A sore that doesn't heal.
2. Nagging cough or hoarseness.
3. Indigestion or difficulty in swallowing.
4. Obvious change in wart or mole.
5. Thickening or lump in breast or elsewhere.
6. Change in bowel or bladder habits.
7. Unusual bleeding or discharge.
If you have any of these symptoms, please visit our clinic immediately.

Phone: 231417 for a free cancer check-up.

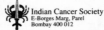

Indian Cancer Society
E-Borges Marg, Parel
Bombay 400 012

O&M/3756

Don't delay your cancer check-up this year. The lives of others depend on it.

Take a little time off today, for someone you love ... and drop in for a cancer check-up. Cancer will strike 5,000 more people in Bombay city alone this year.

The symptoms are so minor at first, you could have cancer and not know it. Yet, our chances of curing cancer are best, when it's detected early. That is why an annual check-up is so important.

Remember ... cancer doesn't always happen to someone else. Get a free check-up at any one of our centres.

Look for these early warning signals of cancer:
1. A sore that doesn't heal.
2. Nagging cough or hoarseness.
3. Indigestion or difficulty in swallowing.
4. Obvious change in wart or mole.
5. Thickening or lump in breast or elsewhere.
6. Change in bowel or bladder habits.
7. Unusual bleeding or discharge.

If you have any of these symptoms, please visit our clinic immediately.

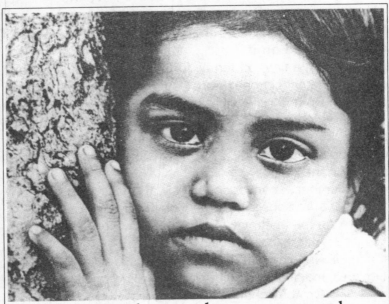

"There's so much we can do to cure cancer today, it's heart-breaking when someone comes too late."

—Dr. D. J. Jussawalla, Indian Cancer Society

Aarti Varma doesn't know the meaning of the word cancer. Yet, it was something that almost changed her life forever.

Aarti's mother had cancer of the womb-- a disease that can be fatal if it is neglected. Today, with the help of modern treatment, Aarti's mother has won her fight against cancer.

"It wasn't luck that saved Mrs. Varma," says Dr. Jussawalla. "It was an early diagnosis.

"Believe me, our chances of curing cancer are more than doubled when it is treated early."

What exactly is cancer?
To put it simply, cancer is the abnormal growth of a body cell. If it is neglected, a cancerous "tumour" can grow very rapidly, and sometimes even spread to other parts of the body.

What are your chances of getting cancer?
Every year, 5,000 more people get cancer in Bombay City alone. Though there are certain high-risk categories, e.g. people who smoke or chew tobacco, just about anyone can get cancer.

How can you tell if you have cancer?
The real tragedy about cancer is that it produces very minor symptoms at first. So you could have cancer, and not know it. The best way to detect cancer, is to come in for a regular yearly check-up.

Is cancer curable?
We've learnt a lot about how to control cancer in recent years. Today, most common cancers are curable, if they're treated early.

Is cancer a frightening disease?
Only if you neglect it. Today, a lot of people are not only winning their fight against cancer, they are even able to lead normal, active lives.

Can you prevent cancer?
You can't really prevent cancer, any more than you can prevent a cold. What you can do is look for any early warning signal, and most important, come in for a regular, annual check-up.

Please, Don't delay your check-up this year. Your life depends on it.

Indian Cancer Society
E-Borges Marg, Parel, Bombay 400 012

Phone: 231417 for a free cancer check-up.

"There's so much we can do to cure cancer today, it's heart-breaking when someone comes too late."
—Dr. D.J.Jussawalla, Indian Cancer Society
Aarti Varma doesn't know the meaning of cancer. Yet, it was something that almost changed her life forever.

Aarti's mother had cancer of the womb — a disease that can be fatal if it is neglected. Today, with the help of modern treatment Aarti's mother has won her fight against cancer.

"It wasn't luck that saved Mrs Varma," says Dr. Jussawalla. "It was an early diagnosis."

"Believe me our chances of curing cancer are more than doubled when it is treated early."

What exactly is cancer?

To put it simply, cancer is the abnormal growth of a body cell. If it is neglected, a cancerous "tumor" can grow very rapidly, and sometimes spread to other parts of the body.

What are you chances of getting cancer?

Every year 5,000 more people get cancer in Bombay city alone. Though there are certain high-risk categories, e.g. people who smoke or chew tobacco, just about anyone can get cancer.

How can you tell if you have cancer?

The real tragedy about cancer is that it produces very minor symptoms at first. So you could have cancer, and not know it. The best way to detect cancer, is to come in for a regular yearly check-up.

Is cancer curable?

We've learned a lot about how to control cancer in recent years. Today, most common cancers are curable, it they're treated early.

Is cancer a frightening disease?

You can't really prevent cancer, any more than you can prevent a cold. What you can do is look for any early warning signal, and most important, come in for a regular, annual check-up.

Please. Don't delay your check-up this year. Your life depends on it.

CANCER REVISITED

Living with cancer the second time was a totally different experience. I was due for my six-monthly check-up that included a CT scan of the chest, a bone scan and an ultrasound of the abdomen. When the results came, the latter two were clear, but the results of the CT scan showed a significant growth in the patch area as compared to the earlier report. I was thunderstruck and once again hoped against hope that there had been some human error in the scan report.

But that was not to be. A new chemotherapy protocol was devised. A new set of drugs, Gemcite and Venelbine, was prescribed. I rushed the scan results to Dr. Advani at the Tata Memorial for a second opinion. He agreed with my oncologists at Batra Hospital and soon, within a week, my chemo-port was working overtime. Each cycle was of three weeks duration, with both drugs repeated on day 1 and day 8 of the cycle.

In my scheme of things, this was a more difficult protocol than the earlier one I had been through. Though the drugs were Level 2 drugs and were known to have less toxic side effects, I had hardly been given any breathing space. As per my previous experience, the seven-day gap between the two stages of the drug administration was just about sufficient time for me to recover from the side effects. And this meant that for about two weeks in each cycle, I would be fighting the side effects and had only about one 'clear' week of no side effects before it was time for the drugs to be repeated again. I felt frightened, wondering whether I would be able to cope with such a strict protocol, especially since my situation was not the same as it was when I last underwent treatment.

My life had changed. I had begun to enjoy my cancer-free days, little realizing that, towards the latter stages, cancer had been steadily gaining ground. My oncologists had warned me that chances of the malignancy recurring were extremely high. They had anticipated that I would need treatment again within six to eight months. It was precisely for this reason that my chemo-port had not been removed. The tests that had been performed at the end of my earlier treatment had confirmed a 95% probability of the absence of cancer. This was the best that medical science offered the world over. Rightly or wrongly, in my own wisdom I had decided that I was in remission. That a near miracle had occurred and I had been rid of the disease.

Lung cancer, in the advanced stage that I was in, has no cure. Only control of the disease is possible with chemotherapy. Patients have been known to undergo many rounds of chemotherapy, which at best have added some years to their life. I had reached Round 2 of my treatment. And like before, my life was turned upside down. Not just mine, but the lives of everyone else around me. My family and my friends. They too would be forced to share my pain and discomfort.

I had taken the initial news bravely. Amrita was with me when the critical tests were done. Our first reaction was that together we would tide this over. As we had done earlier. The medical options were explained, and the final decision was left to us. There were only two possibilities. Either I could ignore the CT scan results and take palliative treatment as and when the cancer symptoms surfaced. Or since I was asymptomatic, chemotherapy could be administered as soon as possible to fight the disease. I was told that chances of disease control were now far lower than the first time round. It was my cancer, my risk, and my decision. Even Dr. Advani's response was mixed. Initially he felt I should go for the first option, but after re-analyzing the situation, recommended at least three rounds of chemotherapy.

There were so many things to consider. How would my treatment interfere with my work schedule? My oncologists had no answers. I had heard of cases, especially in the USA and UK, where patients were able to cope with both their work and treatment schedules. All I could do was hope that the side effects of the drugs would not be severe. The two drugs were known to cause bone marrow suppression that would lead to low blood counts. I had been prone to low blood counts even during the earlier treatment. This frightened me and memories of endless nights at the hospital fighting low blood counts haunted me.

I was also extremely worried about hair loss. I just couldn't picture myself at the office without hair on my head. I went into deep depression about my hair even before the treatment started. Amrita realized what was troubling me. She showed me photographs of my bald head, taken when I was undergoing the earlier treatment. She had even gone to extent of having computer-corrected the same photographs by including the hair on my head. Looking at the two sets of photographs we laughed. She explained to me how my depression about my possible hair-loss was totally baseless.

The new set of drugs had an extremely low possibility of total loss of hair. Besides, even if it were to happen, it could easily be remedied by wearing a wig.

In my period of remission, I had tried to live as normal a life as was possible. However, I couldn't prevent myself from thinking that I had been given a new lease of life. I had heard of people who had survived 15 to 20 years after their treatment and had died a natural and peaceful death. I was not very comfortable at being labeled a cancer survivor. Why was I being called a cancer survivor? Would I continue to be associated with the stigma of cancer for the rest of my life? This had bothered me. Heart patients are not labeled heart attack survivors. Neither are patients who have survived one or another form of a life-threatening ailment. In the beginning, more often than not, at any party that I attended, conversation always shifted to my cancer experiences. I too was guilty since I enjoyed the attention that I received. Soon I realized all this had to stop. I had to concentrate on the tasks at hand rather than continue to think about my cancer. I had to move on. Rehabilitation in society was of prime importance and was taking a longer period than I had anticipated. Maybe this was because the cancer tell-tale signs were evident. The baldness. Or that my confidence levels were extremely low. Whatever the reasons were, I owed it to myself to muster up courage and inner strength so as to once again make significant contributions to society.

All this was of no consequence any more. From being a cancer survivor, I was once again a cancer patient. In a short period of a week, between the diagnosis and the day that Gemcite and Venelbine flowed through my chemo-port, I had to reorient myself to a new way of life. Earlier, I had been given more than six weeks to prepare myself for the chemotherapy treatment. Now, in this short period, I had to be ready to face a new set of challenges. I was certain that some of them would be similar to the ones I had experienced before. And that I would overcome them. Emerge victorious. As I had about 15 months ago.

Today, four cycles have been completed and nearly three months have elapsed. I still don't know whether the cancer in my lungs is responding to the chemotherapy treatment. The critical CT scan was postponed to the beginning of the fifth cycle. I have been through most of the side effects that I had encountered earlier. And more. The nausea, the foul taste in the mouth, the intermittent diarrhea and constipation, the loss of appetite, the tiredness and exhaustion, the shivering, the low blood counts, ... Most of this I was familiar with. Most of this I had experienced earlier.

It was the new side effects of the treatment that frightened me. Even my oncologists did not have the answers to some of them. During my second and third cycle, I developed a low-grade fever. Once a day, my body temperature hovered around 99°C to 100°C and was brought to normal by suitable medication. Initially I ignored the fever. After some days I started feeling weak and breathless. I decided to take leave from work and move to hospital to be under observation and get some tests done. The tests too did not lead to any conclusion. Various theories to explain my low-grade fever were slowly ruled out. The possibility that it was due to some infection in the system or to the cancer or the strong doses of the treatment. As more and more tests were conducted, all these possibilities were ruled out. Finally the doctors concluded that my low-grade fever was a result of the fact that I was immuno-compromised and that there were large variations in my critical blood parameters. And the only thing to do was to ignore the fever.

Weakness and breathlessness was another aspect that I found difficult to cope with. Maybe I was not being able to get sufficient rest as a result of the full day at work. Maybe the chemotherapy protocol, even though Level 2 drugs were being used, was extremely tough and cruel on the system. Maybe it was the fact of my being highly immuno-compromised. Maybe it was just the fact that I was now two years older. Maybe it was a combination of the above and more that was making me weak and breathless. It wasn't as if it was impossible to cope. Every time I felt weak and breathless, all I had to do was some deep-breathing exercises. And in no time I was back in shape. My days started and ended focusing on my treatment. Building a positive attitude and strengthening the mind-body continuum through long hours of meditation and chanting. And in between, I coped with pressures at the office. After office hours I became a recluse. Most times when anyone came to visit me, I felt a desire to leave the room so that I could rest in the peace and quiet of my room. The regular flow of visitors and conversation exhausted me. In the three months since the treatment began, I have not stepped out of the house except to go to the office or the hospital. I have not been able to cope with anything else other than my treatment and office.

At the end of the first cycle, my wisdom tooth started giving me trouble. I was in acute pain and at times I couldn't sleep. I lived on pain-killers. I had painful sensations whenever anything hot and cold touched the right side of my jaw and soon the pain started shooting up towards my head. It was at this stage that I decided to see my dentist. Just before the appointment I happened to mention my dental problem to my oncologist. He was furious, his immediate reaction being that I should cancel the appointment. When I explained to him that the pain was excruciating and unbearable, he warned of dire consequences if I caught any infection at the dentist's clinic. He would not allow the dentist to even touch my teeth with any of his instruments. The question of going any further like filling of a cavity, a root canal or tooth extraction did not arise.

I was shattered and stunned. How could I bear such excruciating pain for the next three to four months? Aren't doctors human? In the end I didn't cancel my visit. After examining my teeth, my dentist concluded that there was a huge cavity in one of my wisdom teeth and that immediate extraction was necessary. There were some other teeth that needed fillings too and if they weren't treated soon might need root canals. All this depressed me further and sitting on the dentist's chair I begged him to find an alternative option to relieve me of my pain. In the end, without any drilling, he filled all my cavities and hoped and prayed that the fillings would stay in position till my chemotherapy was over. Mercifully the pain subsided soon after. Thus far the fillings have helped and apart from the occasional discomfort, the pain has not surfaced as before.

The variable blood counts was another side effect that caused me considerable anxiety. The total leukocyte count (TLC) of the blood was the major culprit. The normal range is 4,000 to 11,000. In my case it fluctuated between 1,000 to over 21,000. At the lower level, I was extremely prone to infection, was put on a course of antibiotics and not allowed any visitors. The upper levels were the result of the medication that I was given to bring the TLC to normal levels. The body soon began to react to these large and abnormal variations. One outward sign was the low-grade fever. The other was the weakness and breathlessness. According to my oncologists, there was no diet in the world that could prevent the low TLC. It resulted from bone marrow suppression, a cumulative effect of the increasing quantity of chemotherapy drugs. Medication could be given as a prophylactic, but the efficacy of the drugs was not guaranteed to prevent the low counts. Once I had to be given five injections before the TLC reached the normal level, when on earlier occasions one injection had sufficed.

Earlier, I had only my cancer to worry about and all my efforts were directed at winning the war. Every day was a new and challenging experience. 24 hours a day, seven days a week all my energies were utilized in combating the disease. There were no external pressures. I was the master of my own time, rested when I felt exhausted, rushed to hospital when things weren't going well. Now, the second time around, all my energies were not only concentrated on fighting cancer but the mind-body continuum had to ensure that I rose above all the side effects of the treatment and was fit enough to cope with the pressures of office.

I was at office six days a week. There were days when work pressures compelled me to stay at office longer. No longer was I able to rest when I was exhausted. Often I had to go against the advice of my doctors who wanted me to be under observation at the hospital. There were days when I was at work with low blood counts and highly prone to infection. I fought nausea at office with high doses of antiemetics, weakness and exhaustion with glucose and a healthy diet, the fever with paracetamols, low blood counts with prophylactic injections. How I managed only I knew. Not skipping a day at work unless it was absolutely essential. The challenges at work became synonymous with those of

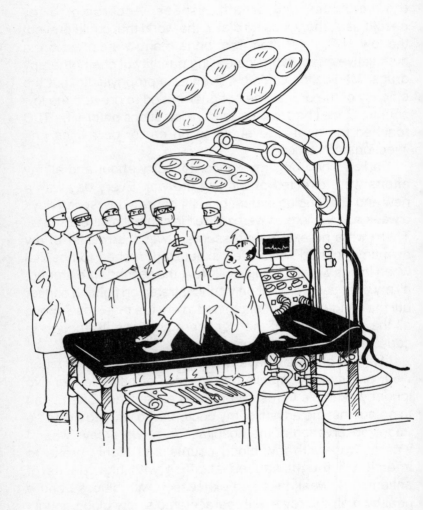

"But how can I tell you are my doctor?"

the treatment. I just had to cope with both.

The recurrence of cancer was perhaps as frightening as the first time when I faced the diagnosis. The 'Why *me*?' syndrome had changed to 'Oh no! not *again.*' But strangely, and in a somewhat convoluted manner, undergoing treatment gave me a sense of security. The fact that something was being done made me feel safe from cancer. During my remission, the absence of any medication or treatment to prevent recurrence had worried me. I felt that nothing was being done to protect me. Now under treatment I felt confident once again and my earlier victory gave me sufficient courage, strength and hope to feel that I would be successful once again.

Be positive and be tough, with a single-minded resolve. Think of the millions of people around the world who have been cancer patients, survived and made significant contributions to society. Integrate the experience of cancer into your life. Never visualize cancer as your enemy, otherwise you will never be able to coexist with it. And be at peace. We all have to deal with our experiences differently and in our own manner. Cancer gives a new meaning to courage, hope, joy and faith. Be proactive and use your experience to help and support others. Cancer has transformed and changed my life. It has redefined aspects of my personality, my career, my goals and the direction the rest of my life will take. It has made me a more complete human being. It has taught me how to cope with the unexpected. It has made me a human being that I am beginning to like.

APPENDICES

1. THE ABC OF CANCER

WHAT IS CANCER?

The organs and tissues of the body are made up of tiny building blocks called cells. Cancer is a disease of these cells. Cells in different parts of the body may look and work differently but they repair and reproduce themselves in the same manner. Normally this division of cells takes place in an orderly and controlled manner, but if for some reason this process gets out of control, the cells develop into a lump called a tumor. The tumor can be benign or malignant. In a benign tumor, the cells do not spread to other parts of the body and so are not cancerous. However, if they continue to grow at the original site they may cause a problem by pressing on the surrounding tissues. A malignant tumor is made up of cancer cells that have the ability to spread beyond the original site and, if left untreated may invade and destroy surrounding tissues. Sometimes, the cells break away from the original (primary) cancer and spread to the other organs in the body via the blood stream or the lymphatic system. When these cells reach a new site they may go on dividing and form a new tumor, often referred to as a 'secondary' or 'metastasis'.

Doctors are able to confirm whether a tumor is benign or malignant by examining a small sample of cells under a microscope. It is important to realize that cancer is not a single disease with a single cause and a single type of treatment. There are more than 200 types of cancer, each with its own name and treatment.

WHAT CAUSES CANCER?

90% of cancers develop because of complex interactions between our bodies, our lifestyles, our genetic make-up and our environment. Tobacco is estimated to cause 30% of all cancer deaths, poor diet 35%, reproductive and sexual behavior 7%, work-related causes 4% and the environment itself 3%. Scientists believe that genetic changes are the basic cause of cancer. Some theories do suggest that cancer may be a hereditary disease because each individual's make-up may make him more susceptible to certain cancers. About 50 of the more than 200 different types of cancer occasionally run in families.

Most of the current scientific evidence indicates that a normal cell is transformed into a cancer cell when certain genes become activated. Recent work in cancer biology concerns the study of oncogenes, a specific gene that participates in changing a normal cell into a cancer cell. It is thought that an oncogene might be present in an inactive form in normal cells and is in some way activated to create cancer cells.

The nature of a person's work or the working environment can also be a factor in developing cancer. For instance exposure to ultraviolet rays in the case of farmers and sailors can lead to certain types of skin cancers; underground miners who get exposed to radon are susceptible to lung cancer as are those people who work with asbestos; workers who use glue, varnishes, etc. are prone to leukemia. Cancers of the lung, breast, prostate and colon and rectum have all become more frequent where risk factors such as cigarette smoking, unhealthy dietary habits and exposure to dangerous chemicals at work or in the environment are now more common. As industrialization has proliferated, so too have the suspected causes of cancer. In recent years, even modern conveniences like pharmaceuticals and cellular telephones have been found to be causes of cancer.

Cancer seems to arise from the effects of two different kinds of cancer-causing agents, or carcinogens. One of these categories comprises agents that damage genes involved in controlling cell proliferation and migration. Cancer arises when a single cell accumulates a number of these mutations, usually over many years, and finally escapes from most restraints on proliferation. The mutations allow the cell and its descendants to develop additional alterations and to accumulate in increasingly large numbers, forming a tumor that consists mostly of these abnormal cells. Another category includes agents that do not damage genes but instead selectively enhance the growth of tumor cells or their precursors. The primary danger of malignancies is that they can metastasize, allowing some of their cells to migrate and thus carry the disease to other parts of the body. Finally, the illness can reach and disrupt one of the body's vital organs.

Smoking, mainly of cigarettes, causes cancer of the lung, upper respiratory tract, esophagus, bladder and pancreas and probably of the stomach, liver and kidney. Whether smoking will result in malignancy depends on several factors including the frequency of smoking, the cigarettes' tar content and, most importantly, the duration of the habit. The risks vary from one type of cancer to another; thus, on average, smokers are twice as likely to be afflicted with cancer of the bladder but eight times more likely to contract cancer of the lung. Passive smoking also causes lung cancer and is as much a killer as general outdoor air pollution or household exposure to the radioactive gas radon.

Obesity in adult life causes cancer of the endometrium (the lining of the uterus) and is an established but relatively weak cause of postmenopausal breast cancer. For unknown reasons, obesity also appears to increase the risk for cancers of the colon, kidney and gall bladder.

Consumption of large quantities of alcoholic beverages, particularly by smokers, increases the risk of cancer of the upper respiratory and digestive tracts, and alcoholic cirrhosis frequently leads to liver cancer. Although modest drinking does seem to reduce the risk of heart disease, recent studies indicate that the intake of as few as one or two drinks a day may contribute to breast and perhaps colon and rectal cancer.

DIFFERENT TYPES OF CANCER

Cancer tumors are named after the part of the body where the cancer first began, and the name does not change even if the cancer spreads to another part of the body. For example, if lung cancer spreads to the breast, it is still classified as lung cancer. Different types of cancer vary in their signs and symptoms, in their growth rate, the manner in which they spread and how they react to different treatments. This is why it is so important to quickly and accurately diagnose cancer, so that specialized treatment can begin immediately. Of the more than 200 different types of cancer, most are distinctly different diseases.

Cancer staging systems describe how far the cancer has spread anatomically. The concept of stage is applicable to almost all cancers except for most forms of leukemia. Since leukemia involves all of the blood, and is not anatomically localized like other cancers, the concept of staging doesn't make as much sense. A few forms of leukemia do have staging systems that reflect various measures of how advanced the disease is.

Cancer is grouped into four stages denoted by Roman numerals I through IV. In general, stage I cancers are small localized cancers that are usually curable, while stage IV usually represents inoperable or metastatic cancer. Stage II and III cancers are usually locally advanced and with the involvement of local lymph nodes. These stages are defined precisely but the definition is different for each kind of cancer. In addition, it is important to realize that the prognosis for a given stage also depends on what kind of cancer it is, so that a stage II non-small-cell lung cancer has a different prognosis from a stage II cervical cancer.

Unfortunately, it is common for cancer to return months or years after the primary tumor has been removed. This is because cancer cells might have already broken away and lodged in distant locations by the time the primary tumor was discovered, but had not formed tumors which were large enough to be detected at that time. Sometimes a tiny bit of the primary tumor is left behind in the initial surgery and this later grows into a macroscopic tumor. Cancer that recurs after the visible tumor has been eradicated is called 'recurrent disease'.

For many cancers four prognostic groups are not enough, so the overall staging is further divided with classifications like IIa, and IIb. People assume that the differences in prognosis between sub-groups, like IIIa and IIIb, is smaller than between major divisions like II and III, but this is not necessarily the case. For instance, in non-small-cell lung cancer, the difference between stage IIIa and stage IIIb is very significant. People with stage IIIa cancer have a chance of being cured with treatment that includes surgery, whereas surgery generally does not help people at stage IIIb who have a substantially worse prognosis.

SIGNS AND SYMPTOMS OF CANCER

Since prevention is one of the most important cancer-fighting tools, it is critical that cancer be detected as early as possible before it spreads. Tell-tale signs of cancer include a lump or thickening in the breast or testicles; a change in a wart or mole; a skin sore or a persistent sore throat that doesn't heal; a change in bowel or bladder habits; a persistent cough or the coughing of blood; constant indigestion or trouble in swallowing; unusual bleeding or vaginal discharge; and chronic fatigue.

The following are symptoms that may occur in specific types of cancers:

Bladder cancer: Blood in the urine, pain or burning upon urination; frequent urination; or cloudy urine.

Bone cancer: Pain in the bone or swelling around the affected site; fractures in bones; weakness, fatigue; weight loss; repeated infections; nausea, vomiting, constipation, problems with urination; weakness or numbness in the legs; or bumps and bruises that persist.

Brain cancer: Dizziness; drowsiness; abnormal eye movements or changes in vision; weakness, loss of feeling in arms or legs or difficulties in walking; fits or convulsions; changes in personality, memory or speech; or headaches that tend to be worse in the morning and ease during the day, that may be accompanied by nausea or vomiting.

Breast cancer: A lump or thickening of the breast; discharge from the nipple; change in the skin of the breast; a feeling of heat; or enlarged lymph nodes under the arm.

Colorectal cancer: Rectal bleeding (red blood in stools, or black stools); abdominal cramps; constipation alternating with diarrhea; weight loss; loss of appetite; weakness; or pallid complexion.

Kidney cancer: Blood in urine; dull ache or pain in the back or side; or lump in kidney area, sometimes accompanied by high blood pressure or abnormality in red blood cell count.

Leukemia: Weakness, paleness; fever and flu-like symptoms; bruising and prolonged bleeding; enlarged lymph nodes, spleen, liver; pain in bones and joints; frequent infections; weight loss; or night sweats.

Lung cancer: Wheezing, persistent cough for months; blood-streaked sputum; persistent ache in chest; congestion in lungs; or enlarged lymph nodes in the neck.

Melanoma: Change in mole or other bump on the skin, including bleeding or change in size, shape, color, or texture.

Non-Hodgkin's lymphoma: Painless swelling in the lymph nodes in the neck, underarm, or groin; persistent fever; feeling of fatigue; unexplained weight loss; itchy skin and rashes; small lumps in skin; bone pain; swelling in the abdomen; or liver or spleen enlargement.

Oral cancer: A lump in the mouth, ulceration of the lip, tongue or inside of the mouth that does not heal within a couple of weeks; dentures that no longer fit well; or oral pain, bleeding, foul breath, loose teeth, and changes in speech.

Ovarian cancer: Abdominal swelling; in rare cases, abnormal vaginal bleeding; or digestive discomfort.

Pancreatic cancer: Upper abdominal pain and unexplained weight loss; pain near the center of the back; intolerance of fatty foods; yellowing of the skin; abdominal masses; or enlargement of liver and spleen.

Prostate cancer: Urination difficulties due to blockage of the urethra; urine retention, creating frequent feelings of urgency to urinate, especially at night; burning or painful urination; bloody urine; tenderness over the bladder; or dull ache in the pelvis or back.

Stomach cancer: Indigestion or heartburn; discomfort or pain in the abdomen; nausea and vomiting; diarrhea or constipation; bloating after meals; loss of appetite; weakness and fatigue; or bleeding and vomiting blood or blood in the stool.

Uterine cancer: Abnormal vaginal bleeding, watery bloody discharge in postmenopausal women; painful urination; pain during intercourse; or pain in pelvic area.

THE DIAGNOSIS

If you have a sign or symptom that might mean you have cancer, the doctor will do a physical examination and ask about your medical history. Typically, various tests and examinations will be ordered. They may include imaging procedures, which produce pictures of areas inside the body; or the use of various scopes, which allows the doctor to look directly inside certain organs; and laboratory tests.

One of the most important investigations is the physical examination done by the surgeon or oncologist. Your lungs, liver, abdomen, back and limbs will be examined for abnormalities. Your breast may be examined and any lumps will be measured. Your armpit and neck will be felt to see if any lymph nodes are enlarged. Not all enlarged lymph nodes are cancerous: the doctor will try to determine this by assessing whether a node feels normal or enlarged, soft or hard, and whether it is movable. If a suspicious lymph node is found, a fine-needle biopsy will probably be done. Blood tests will be done to check whether your bone marrow, liver and kidneys are working normally.

Most specialists also order a chest x-ray to check the condition of the lungs and to ascertain the presence of any benign or malignant lung disease. For older patients, an electrocardiogram (ECG) may be done to check the heart. A bone scan is only necessary for patients who have a high risk of metastasis to the bones or actual symptoms of such metastasis. The same goes for ultrasound examinations of the liver. If liver metastasis is highly unlikely then an ultrasound is not done routinely.

Images of areas inside the body help the doctor tell whether a tumor is present. These images can be made in several ways. In many cases, a special dye is used so that certain organs show up better on film. The dye may be swallowed or put into the body through a needle or tube. An x-ray is the most common method used by doctors to take pictures of the inside of the body. In a special kind of x-ray imaging, a CT or CAT scan uses a computer connected to an x-ray machine to make a series of detailed pictures. In radio-nuclide scanning, the patient swallows or is given an injection of a mildly radioactive substance. A machine (scanner) measures radioactivity levels in certain organs and prints a picture on paper or film and by looking at the amount of radioactivity in the organs, the doctor can find the abnormal areas.

Ultrasonography is another procedure for viewing the inside of the body. High-frequency sound waves that cannot be heard by humans enter the body and bounce back. Their echoes produce a picture called a sonogram. These pictures are shown on a monitor like a TV screen and can be printed on paper. In an MRI, also known as Magnetic Resonance Imaging, a powerful magnet is linked to a computer to make detailed pictures of areas in the body. These pictures are viewed on a monitor and can also be printed.

Endoscopy, bronchoscopy, and colonoscopy allow the doctor to look into the body through a lighted tube. The examination is named after the organ involved. For example, a colonoscopy looks inside the colon. During the examination, the doctor may collect tissue or cells for closer examination and laboratory testing.

No single test can diagnose cancer, but laboratory tests give doctors important information. If cancer is present, these tests may show the effects of the disease on the body. In some cases, special tests are used to measure the amount of certain substances in the blood, urine, other body fluids and tumor tissue. The levels of these substances may become abnormal when certain kinds of cancer are present. These tests may also be used to monitor the effects of treatment on the body.

Cancer is also diagnosed by physically removing a sample (tissue, cells, or fluid) of a suspected tumor and examining this material under a microscope. This procedure is called a biopsy. Microscopic examination of biopsy samples is the only way that a definite diagnosis of cancer can be made. After careful evaluation, a benign or malignant diagnosis can usually be established. While these techniques are generally accurate and reliable, situations where the needle misses the tumor can cause the biopsy to appear benign when in fact a cancerous tumor does exist. In this situation, it may be necessary to repeat the biopsy procedure. The material from the tumor is usually removed using a very thin needle attached to a syringe so as to extract (aspirate) individual or small clusters of cells. This technique, called FNAC (Fine Needle Aspiration Cytology) is used alone when the mass can be clearly felt (palpated) through the skin. For subtle or deep lesions that cannot be felt through the skin, this procedure is used along with x-ray, CT or ultrasound guidance.

During surgery, it may be necessary to determine whether a tumor is benign or malignant. A frozen section is a rapid process that allows the pathologist to give the surgeon an on-the-spot diagnosis while the patient is still in the operating room. In this procedure, the surgeon removes a sample of tissue and submits it to the pathologist. Microscopic slides are then prepared and examined by the pathologist. The entire procedure takes 10-12 minutes. The pathologist discusses his findings with the surgeon who can then determine the best surgical procedure to perform.

PAP smears are routinely used to examine cells from the surface of the cervix. In this procedure, the surface of the cervix is scraped with a spatula-shaped instrument to obtain a sample of cells. These cells are then stained and examined under a microscope by a pathologist who makes a diagnosis.

If the above tests confirm the cancer, it is necessary to perform other tests to see whether there has been any spread of the disease to other parts of the body. The results of these tests help in deciding the treatment best suited in the individual's case:

CT scan: It is necessary to study the CT scan images of the abdomen and the head so as to rule out any metastasis in these parts of the body.

Liver and/or abdomen ultrasound: In this test, sound waves are used to make a complete picture of the area. This is used to measure the size and position of a tumor if it exists in this region. A liver isotope scan is also done if any abnormality is detected in the ultrasound test.

Bone scan: A mild radioactive substance is injected into a vein, and a scan taken about two to four hours later. More radioactivity goes to the abnormal than the normal bone, and these areas get picked up by the scanner, so as to highlight any bone metastasis.

THE TREATMENT

Surgery, radiotherapy and chemotherapy may be used alone or together to treat cancer. The mode of treatment takes into account the results of all the earlier tests, as also the age, general health, the type and size of tumor, what it looks like under the microscope and whether it has spread beyond the primary region. Two teams of doctors can have different views about the specific treatment to be followed.

Surgery: This is often used to treat cancer when there is no spread or limited spread. The type of operation chosen would depend upon the size and position of the tumor. Surgery is not generally used to treat cancer that is not localized. It can take several weeks to recover from surgery, although some patients recover more quickly than others do.

Radiotherapy: This treats cancer by using high-energy rays that destroy the cancer cells, while doing as little harm as possible to normal cells. It can be used alone or after surgery to treat all types of cancers. The length of the treatment is dependent upon the type and size of the cancer. Treatment planning is a very important part of radiotherapy and can take several visits to the radiotherapist. Radiotherapy is not painful but you need to be still for a few minutes while your treatment is being administered.

Chemotherapy: This uses special anti-cancer (cytotoxic) drugs to destroy the cancer cells. These drugs work by disrupting the growth of cancer cells and are most commonly used for cancers in which metastasis has been identified. The drugs are sometimes given as tablets or, more usually intravenously. Chemotherapy is given as a course of treatment lasting a few days, followed by a period of rest of a few weeks which allows the body to recover from any side effects of the treatment. The number of cycles of treatment depends on the type of cancer and the response to the drugs.

2. THE SIDE EFFECTS OF CHEMOTHERAPY

The side effects of anti-cancer treatment, especially chemotherapy, can be unpleasant, but they must be measured against the treatment's ability to destroy cancer. People undergoing chemotherapy treatment can get discouraged about the length of time the treatment is taking, the costs and the side effects. Because cancer cells grow and divide rapidly, these drugs are designed to kill fast-growing cells. There are normal, healthy cells that also multiply quickly and the chemotherapy drugs can also affect these cells, resulting in side effects.

The fast growing, normal cells most likely to get affected are blood-forming cells in the bone marrow and cells in the digestive tract, reproductive system and hair follicles. Some chemotherapy drugs can also damage cells of the heart, kidney, bladder, lungs and the nervous system. Whether you have a particular side effect and how severe it will be, depends on the kind of chemotherapy being administered and how the body reacts to it. Most normal cells recover quickly after the chemotherapy is over, and most side effects gradually disappear after the treatment ends and the healthy cells have a chance to grow normally. Besides, newer and better medicines are available to control the extent of discomfort and damage arising from the treatment. While many side effects go away fairly rapidly, certain ones may take months or years to disappear completely. It is, however, important to remember that many people have no long-term problems as a result of chemotherapy.

Some of the side effects of chemotherapy include:

Nausea and vomiting: Chemotherapy can cause nausea and vomiting by affecting the stomach, the area of the brain that controls vomiting or both. The reaction varies from person to person and from drug to drug, and can last from a few hours after the treatment to a few days. Nausea and vomiting can almost always be controlled or lessened using a range of drugs known as antiemetics.

Hair loss: Hair loss is a common side effect of chemotherapy and can lead to hair becoming thinner or falling totally. Hair loss can occur on all parts of the body, not just the head. Facial hair, arm and leg hair, underarm hair and pubic hair may get affected. The hair usually grows back after the treatment is over.

Fatigue and anemia: Chemotherapy can reduce the bone marrow's ability to produce red blood cells which carry oxygen to all parts of the body. And when the red blood cells get reduced, the body tissues don't get enough oxygen to do their work. This condition is called anemia and can make a patient feel very tired and weak. Regular blood tests are essential during the treatment and corrective action can be taken either through a blood transfusion or injections.

Infections: Chemotherapy can also affect the bone marrow and reduce its ability to produce white blood cells which are required to fight many types of infections. An infection can begin from any part of the body including the mouth, skin, lungs, urinary tract, rectum and reproductive tract. Regular blood tests during the treatment ensure that remedial action can be taken in any situation.

Blood clotting problems: Chemotherapy can also affect the bone marrow's ability to produce platelets, the blood cells that help stop bleeding by making your blood clot. The absence of the required level of platelets may lead to bleeding or bruising more easily, even from a minor injury. Regular monitoring of the platelet count is essential with blood tests, and a blood transplant may be required to build up the count.

Mouth, gum and throat problems: Anti-cancer drugs can cause sores and ulcers in the mouth and throat. They can also make these tissues dry and irritated or cause them to bleed. This can be prevented through careful personal hygiene and medication when necessary.

Diarrhea: Cells lining the intestine can also get affected, resulting in diarrhea. Medication is available to bring it under control.

Constipation: Some anti-cancer drugs can lead to constipation and the use of laxatives may be necessary.

Nerve and muscle effects: The nervous system affects just about every organ and tissue of the body. So when chemotherapy affects the cells of the nervous system as the drugs sometimes do, a wide range of side effects can result. Certain drugs can cause peripheral neuropathy, a condition that can make you feel a tingling, burning, weakness, or numbness in the hands and/or feet. Other symptoms include loss of balance, clumsiness, difficulty in picking up objects, walking problems, jaw pain, hearing loss and weakening of muscles. In some cases the nerve and muscle effects may not be serious and in other cases these symptoms can lead to serious problems that need medical attention.

Effects on skin and nails: Possible side effects on the

skin include redness, itching, peeling, dryness and acne. The nails may become brittle, darkened or cracked and may even develop vertical lines or bands. Most of these skin problems are not serious and are reversible after the treatment is completed.

Kidney and bladder effects: Some anti-cancer drugs can irritate the bladder or cause temporary or permanent damage to the kidneys. This can lead to pain or burning during passing of urine, frequent urination, reddish or bloody urine, and even fever and chills. Plenty of fluid intake can prevent these problems.

Flu-like syndrome: Some patients report feeling as though they have the flu a few hours in the day after chemotherapy. Flu-like symptoms including muscle ache, headache, tiredness, slight fever, chill and poor appetite can last up to three days and can be caused by an infection or the cancer itself.

Fluid retention: Your body may retain excessive fluids as a result of hormonal changes from the therapy. If the problem is severe, the doctor may prescribe medication to get rid of the extra fluids.

Sexual effects: Chemotherapy can, but does not always, effect sexual organs and their functioning. The side effects that might occur depend on the drugs used and the person's age and general health. Amongst men, anti-cancer drugs may lower the number of sperm cells or cause other abnormalities that can result in temporary or permanent infertility. This does not, however, affect the ability to have sexual intercourse. Amongst women, anti-cancer drugs can damage the ovaries and reduce the amount of hormones they produce. As a result, the menstrual periods can become irregular or stop completely during chemotherapy. These hormonal effects may cause menopause-like symptoms such as hot flushes, itching, burning or dryness of the vaginal tissues. Damage to the ovaries can lead to temporary or permanent infertility and the inability to become pregnant. Pregnancy, though possible, is not advisable since some anti-cancer drugs may cause birth defects. If a woman is pregnant when her cancer is discovered, it may be necessary to delay chemotherapy until after the baby is born or start it after the 12th week of pregnancy, when the fetus is beyond the stage of greatest risk. In some cases termination of the pregnancy may also be necessary.

3. PRECAUTIONS YOU SHOULD TAKE DURING TREATMENT

Most of the side effects mentioned earlier may or may not occur and are dependent on the drugs used and the general health condition of the patient. Usually doctors are able to suggest ways to reduce the side effects or make them easier to be tolerated. They can be controlled through additional medication. It is important that your doctor is made aware of any symptoms or changes in your body and his advice followed so that preventive action can be taken as and when necessary.

Chemotherapy can also bring about major changes in a person's life. It can affect overall health, threaten a sense of well-being, disrupt day-to-day schedules and put a strain on personal relationships. Patients can feel fearful, anxious, angry or depressed at the same moment. These emotions are perfectly normal and understandable, but can be very disturbing. The best way to cope with these emotions and stress resulting from cancer and its treatment is to ensure that the mind and body are fighting the war together.

Some of the precautions that should be taken during chemotherapy are listed here:

CARE OF HAIR:

Use mild shampoos.

Use a soft hair brush and comb.

Don't use brush rollers to set your hair.

Don't dye your hair.

Have your hair cut short.

Use a cap or scarf or a wig to protect your scalp from the sun if you lose a lot of hair on your head.

PREVENTION OF FATIGUE:

Get plenty of rest, sleep longer hours at night and take naps during the day.

Limit your activities and do the things that are the most important.

Don't be afraid to ask for help when you need it.

Eat a well-balanced diet.

When sitting or lying down, get up slowly to prevent dizziness.

PREVENTION OF INFECTIONS:

Wash your hands often during the day, especially before eating.

Clean your rectal area gently but thoroughly after using the toilet.

Stay away from people who have diseases you can catch like colds, the flu, measles, chickenpox, etc.

Avoid crowds.

Stay away from children who have recently received immunization.

Don't cut or tear the cuticles of your nails.

Be careful not to cut or nick yourself when using scissors, needles or knives, or during shaving.

Use a soft toothbrush that won't hurt your gums.

Don't squeeze or scratch pimples.

Take a warm bath daily, dry your skin softly without rigorous rubbing.

Use lotion or oil to soften or heal your skin if it becomes dry or cracked.

Clean cuts and scrapes right away with warm water, soap and antiseptic.

Be alert to the signs that indicate infection including fever over 100 degrees F; chills; sweating; loose bowels; a burning feeling during urination; a cough or a sore throat; unusual vaginal discharge or itching; redness or swelling around a wound or sore.

Pay special attention to your eyes, nose, mouth, genital and rectal areas.

BLEEDING:

Don't take any medicines without the doctor's advice.

Don't drink alcoholic beverages.

Use a very soft toothbrush.

Clean your nose gently with a soft tissue.

Prevent cuts and nicks while shaving or using scissors.

Be careful not to burn yourself while cooking or ironing.

Avoid sports or other activities that might lead to injury.

CARE OF MOUTH:

Good oral care is essential to prevent sores and ulcers in the mouth and throat.

If possible consult your dentist before you begin chemotherapy to ensure that there are no dental problems like cavities, etc.

Brush your teeth and gums after every meal using a soft toothbrush.

Rinse the toothbrush well after each use and store in a

dry place.
>Use a mild mouthwash if necessary.
>Drink lots of fluids during and after chemotherapy.

4. THE FUTURE OF CANCER TREATMENT

The initial impact of major breakthroughs in cancer treatment is still being felt, but mainly in research laboratories. Gene therapy is still in its early infancy; concepts of protein therapy are being tested; and though some advances in laser therapy are now available for cancer patients, a lot of development work is still being undertaken. Oncologists are not yet looking at all these therapies as a cure for cancer, but rather as a proof of new interventions in the future and the first step toward a new generation of cancer treatment. Gene therapy encompasses the deliberate alteration of the genetic material of cancer cells. It involves the administration of living cells that have been genetically manipulated or processed so as to change their biological characteristics. Current approaches to delivering genes into cells include physico-chemical methods, viral vectors and direct DNA injections. Attempts have been made to replace the inactivated, tumor-suppressor genes in cancer cells. However, the snag is that cancer cells comprise several, if not myriad, mutated genes, and tumor homogeneity does not exist. Repairing all gene mutations in the cancer lesions of a patient is the biggest challenge and the concentration is on the development of 'smart bombs' that will target only the cancer cells and not cause any damage to the normal ones.

A number of drugs are at various stages of development. Herceptin blocks the binding of the growth factors by attacking the receptors on the surface of breast cancer cells. Onyx-015, a virus that works on the cancer cells only, combined with chemotherapy, is proving to be effective even in recurrent, late-stage head and neck cancer. Glivec, a drug that disables the protein produced inside cells of chronic leukemia, is providing spectacular results in its clinical trials. So is Zevalin, an antibody hooked to the radioisotope yttrium-90, testing well amongst Non-Hodgkins lymphoma patients. P-53, a gene being developed, can stop a damaged cell from turning into a cancerous one and can begin to trigger a self-destruction program for the cancer cell. It is indicative of the possibility of restoring a normal functioning gene in a cancer cell. SU5416 targets the receptors in the signal-transduction process; and the anti-VEGF is aimed at a growth factor in the cells. Both these work at vulnerable points somewhere along the lines of communication between cells and attempt to disrupt them.

Gene therapy includes a wide spectrum of interventions. Tumor cells can serve as vehicles to carry therapeutic genes into cancer lesions where the gene product can exert an anti-cancer effect. Over 300 compounds and molecules are being tested on cancer patients, a number of them based on new and hitherto untried ways of attacking tumors. Hundreds more are in early stages of development and gene therapy protocols seem to be a worthy goal in cancer research. However, it seems unlikely that gene therapy will provide magic anti-cancer bullets in the near future or that a definitive cancer cure will emerge before the next 5-10 years. The heart of the cancer cell is being investigated, and the life and death of cells is being analyzed. The molecules in the body that participate in these pathways are now the targets of new therapies. Developments in gene therapy are not only being focused on the destruction of cancer cells or the fixing of what is broken in a cell that is causing the unregulated growth. Efforts are being made to find effective weapons that will interfere with the signals involved in tumor growth.

The prevention of the reproduction of a cancer cell or its self-destruction is being experimented by cutting its communication lines. In order to grow, tumors need nourishment. They need to be fed. Though the actual process is extremely complex, the basic principle is simple. When lines of communication are working properly, they enable cells to perform normal functions and when they breakdown, problems develop. By cutting off the tumor's food supply, it cannot grow. This is the basis of protein therapy. Some signal-jamming treatments use tiny proteins similar to antibodies on the immune system. Or those that bind to the surface of a cancer cell.

Other options under development include the use of radioactive isotope-carrying antibodies which destroy the cancer cells without affecting the surrounding tissues. By injecting cancer patients with a gene that acts to slow down the disease, the growth of cancer tumors can be reduced or even be shrunk. Attempts are also being made to change the genetic code of cancer cells inside the body. This could prove to be the key to treating cancer tumors in the lung, colon and breast. The problem with cancer cells is that they don't know when to quit. The uncontrolled growth of tumors shoves aside healthy tissue, causing pain, debilitation and often, death. The immune response has to be enhanced and stimulated for the current gene therapy approaches to become more successful than the available chemotherapy treatment. This is because it is extremely difficult to target every cancer cell with a gene encoding mechanism of killing the cancer cell and not the normal cell.

Interestingly, one form of gene therapy that is being developed involves the boosting of the immune system. Antibodies are being drafted to prod the immune system into destroying the cancer cells by making the immune system recognize cancer cells as some kind of foreign invaders in the body. Like bacteria and viruses. A number of other gene therapy approaches have been devised and clinical trials designed. The design of an adenovirus that will kill cells that have abnormal suppressor genes and leave unaffected those with normal genes is another direction that gene therapy is investigating. The idea is that the gene would enter into all tumor cells and only kill those with the abnormal gene, i.e. only the cancer cells. This approach by itself is not likely to be as effective as its design would suggest. Most solid tumors diversify and develop several different pathways of abnormality and it is likely that cells will be selected with a different oncogene expression or a different mutant suppressor type. And the solid tumor may develop resistance in a similar manner as it does to chemotherapy.

The therapies being developed may not be able to get rid of large tumors. A combination of treatments, each using a different strategy, may be necessary. Traditional chemotherapy may have to be combined with some of the new developments as and when made available, to force cancer cells to self-destruct. Or stop them from increasing in size. Tumors cannot grow beyond a particular size without an ever-expanding network of blood vessels, and attempts are being made to stop this process. New approaches that complement cancer vaccines are being tested. Attempts to stimulate the immune system in patients has led to a renaissance in tumor immunology, with the realization that all solid tumors have some form of associated antigen or a specific antigen which can be exploited as a target for cancer vaccines. No appropriate adjuvant has been used in most studies when presenting the immune system with a specific antigen. And it is now being found that the right type of immune response has to be invoked. Results from gene therapy studies may probably be slower than the vaccine studies, the latter having the advantages of being practical, being of relatively low cost, and having very few side effects.

Oncologists have now begun to offer a new, non-surgical treatment that uses laser beams to blast cancer cells, after certain drugs have been induced. For instance, for people with lung cancer, the user of laser therapy or photodynamic therapy involves the administration of the FDA-approved drug, Photofrin, which gets absorbed by the tumor in high concentrations. When Photofrin is exposed to light from a cold laser, it destroys the tumor without harming the surrounding tissues. Photodynamic therapy can offer a cure for lung cancer patients whose tumors are still small and confined to the airways. The treatment can also give significant palliative relief to patients with advanced cancer who have difficulty breathing because of tumors that are blocking the airways. In the case of lung cancer, photodynamic therapy offers another option for those who are not candidates for traditional surgery or radiation due to advanced age, frail health, tumors that are too numerous, or other factors. For the treatment, which is performed on an outpatient basis, the patients first receive an intravenous infusion of Photofrin. Over the next 48 hours, the drug becomes concentrated within the tumors. Then the patients come back two days later, and under mild sedation, a bronchoscope within which is inserted a Yag laser that is focused on the tumor, is used. The light activates the Photofrin, which then begins to destroy the tumor. The patients must stay out of the sun for the next four weeks because the treatment puts them at risk of severe sunburn.

It is still too early to declare victory in the war on cancer, since a large number of drugs being developed may or may not pass the clinical trials and get FDA approval. However, there is a new surge of optimism among oncologists. Soon the 'hit and try' methods of cancer treatment will be over. Oncologists would be able to analyze why a set of drugs is not working and would then be in a position to choose from a vast array of other options that would be more effective. What were distant dreams of cancer patients in the last millennium will soon become a reality. The combination of knowledge (or the understanding of the questions to be asked) and technology (or the means of getting the answers) is pushing the success in cancer treatment forward at a swift pace.

5. THE SUPER FOODS

The food we eat is our medicine. The medicine we take is our food. And together they act as our nourishment to fight cancer. One without the other will not help in our final battle. Just as a malignant cell has many pathways, each with its own rules and regulations, so does our food. Our medication. And these are just two of the myriad support systems we use to win the war. Perhaps the most significant of the tools in our possession. Proper nutrition is absolutely essential at all stages of cancer. There are certain foods that help in preventing the onslaught of cancer. Others can help in coping with the many side effects of treatment. And when we recover from cancer, then recovering from the therapy and preventing the recurrence of cancer can be equally, if not even more, challenging. In our diet. Our healthy living. Our medication. And more significantly, for the mind-body continuum.

All round the world, cancer patients and their families have their own stories to tell. In their experiences. In the foods that were used. And the medication. Both during and after the treatment. For instance, in Germany digestive enzymes and mistletoe are government-approved cancer drugs. The leaves and berries of the ginkgo tree contain a wide assortment of curative properties and have been a pivotal medicine in China for over 5,000 years. In England, primrose oil is accepted cancer therapy. For centuries, native South Americans have been making therapeutic use of cat's claw, a woody wine that grows to more than 30 meters by wrapping itself around nearby trees. The bark of the yew tree, Taxol, holds promise as a potent cancer drug. One of the best-selling cancer drugs in the world is a mushroom extract, PSK, manufactured in Japan, and used all over Europe and Japan. Closer home in India, tulsi leaves and water from the holy Ganga are claimed to have immense healing properties.

Eat foods in as close to their natural state as possible. Expand your horizons. Eat a variety of foods so that the healing process is based on the combined nutrients of all foods that are part of your diet. After a lifetime of high fat, high sugar, overeating, too much alcohol, stress, drugs, indigestible foods, cancer patients find that it is not so simple to change to healthy eating. Even to concentrate on the super foods that have proven and accepted properties that help fight cancer. The list below is by no means exhaustive but indicative of the kinds of foods that are beneficial for cancer patients. And the kind of support they can provide in the war against cancer.

Garlic: This highly pungent vegetable has been used for over 5,000 years in various healing processes. Garlic has been found to stimulate natural protection against cancer cells. It provides the liver with some amount of protection against carcinogenic chemicals. And while it attacks the invading specific cells, it is completely harmless on the normal cells, thereby offering hope of a truly selective toxin against cancer.

Carotenoids and bioflavonoids: Both these substances have the potential of stimulating the immune system. Also, carotenoids are believed to be directly toxic to cancer cells. Carotenoids are found in green and orange fruits and vegetables while bioflavonoids are found in citrus fruits, whole grains, honey and other plant foods.

Cruciferous vegetables: Ingredients in vegetables like broccoli, Brussels sprouts, cabbage and cauliflower have been isolated and found to be very protective against cancer. These vegetables are able to increase the body's production of glutathione peroxidase, which is one of the more important protective enzymes of the body.

Mushrooms: Certain types of mushrooms help prevent cancer growth. There is enough evidence to indicate that PSK, Rei-shi, Shiitake and Maitake mushrooms are potent anti-cancer foods. Mushrooms help cancer patients by acting as immune stimulants and reducing the toxic effects of chemotherapy. They also inhibit metastasis and lower excess blood sugar levels and hypertension, apart from providing protection to the liver.

Legumes: Seed foods like soybeans have a substance that partially protects the seed from digestion. For a long time this was considered harmful. Recent studies indicate that this substance has potent anti-cancer properties and can actually prevent cancer when exposed to a variety of carcinogens. It can retard cancer growth, lower the toxic side effects of chemotherapy and radiation therapy and revert cancer cells back to normal, healthy cells.

Green tea: Green tea contains a variety of polyphenolic compounds that work as an antioxidant, even more potent than vitamin C. Studies have indicated that green tea users have about half the cancer incidence as that of non-tea drinkers. It shuts down the specific promoters involved in breast cancer and also inhibits the formation of cancer-causing agents in the stomach. Green tea also acts as an immune stimulant and a metastasis inhibitor.

Tomatoes: Lycopenes, the reddish pigments in tomatoes, and for that matter in watermelon and red grapefruit, are potent antioxidants, immune stimulants and regulators of the cancer gene expression. Studies have indicated that as little as one serving of tomatoes a week can reduce the risk of certain types of cancer, and that the higher the level of lycopenes the lower the incidence of certain cancers.

Ginseng: This is one of the oldest and most widely studied herbs. It helps cancer patients with its ability to bring about biochemical adjustments; lowers blood glucose levels since cancer is a sugar feeder; acts as an immune stimulant; controls cell growth and suppresses abnormal cell division.

Turmeric: The active ingredient in turmeric, and mustard, is a yellow pigment which enhances the immune system by protecting the cells from their own poisons. Amongst patients with skin cancer, turmeric-based ointments provide significant reduction in the itching, pain and size of the lesions.

Vitamin C: This is one of the more versatile vitamins. It stimulates the immune system against cancer; provides protection against free radicals; lowers cancer incidence; enhances the toxicity of chemotherapy and radiation therapy against cancer cells; slows down and even reverses cell degeneration.

Vitamin A: This was one of the first micro-nutrients recognized for its role in preventing cancer. It helps in cell division and cell communication; slows down and/or reverses some forms of cancer; acts as an immune stimulant.

Vitamin E: Because of its fundamental role in cell biology, Vitamin E acts as an immune regulator by protecting immune cells from destruction as they fight cancer. It prevents damage to the skin from ultraviolet radiation; protects against the carcinogenic effects of tobacco; helps cancer treatment to distinguish between healthy and cancerous cells.

Others: There are numerous other foods that have the ability to slow specific growth in some manner. These include apples, apricots, barley, figs, fish, fish oil, ginger, spinach and seaweed.

6. CANCER SOCIETIES
AND HOW THEY CAN HELP YOU

AM CHARITABLE TRUST

128 Kamalapuri Colony, Phase III
Hyderabad 500 073
Andhra Pradesh
Tel: 6580116, 3554304
Fax: 3541733
Website: www.cancerhope.org

Founded in 1998, the Trust provides hope to patients even in advanced stages of cancer. It assists in minimizing pain and suffering caused by chemotherapy/radiotherapy. It also helps in improving the quality of life of patients through alternative scientific approaches and identifying the factors that lead to cure. The Trust scientifically validates alternative therapies, using the most modern and advanced testing techniques and carries out programs for early detection of cancer.

ATHULYA AYURVEDIC MEDICAL RESEARCH CENTRE
Mundikkal Thazham Medical College
Karnthoor Road
Kottamparamba Post
Calicut 670 008
Kerala
Tel: 358016, 356391
Website: www.ayurvediccancertherapy.com

The Medical Research Centre provides cancer therapy using ayurvedic medication. Depending on the response, the patient is advised to take specific supportive therapy also.

CANCER PATIENTS AID ASSOCIATION (CPAA)
Anand Niketan
King George V Memorial
Dr. E Moses Road
Mahalaxmi
Mumbai 400 011
Maharashtra
Tel: 4924000, 4928775
Fax: 4973599
e-mail: webmaster@cpaaindia.org
Website: www.cpaaindia.org

CPAA provides total management of cancer for patients. Its activities encompass raising awareness, early detection, insurance, counseling, medical and financial aid and rehabilitation. The main thrust is on spreading awareness on the dangers inherent in chewing tobacco, early marriage, multiple pregnancies, etc., which are responsible for approximately 70% of cancers in India. It also takes steps for the early detection of cancer.

CANSUPPORT

38 Shahpur Jat, 2nd Floor
New Delhi 110 049
Tel: 6497154, 6497153
e-mail: cansup-india@hotmail.com
Website: www.cansupport-india.org

CanSupport believes that people with cancer and their families deserve the highest quality medical, nursing and psychological care and that everyone has the right to live life to its fullest without pain and to die with dignity. CanSupport's Home Care teams offer support to patients and families and help them experience the highest quality of life possible during the terminal phase of cancer.

COIMBATORE CANCER FOUNDATION
GKNM Hospital
Pappanaicken Palayam
Coimbatore 641 037
Tamil Nadu
Tel: 216211
Fax: 211611
e-mail: cancerfdn@coimbatore.com
Website: www.coimbatore.com/cancerfdn/ccf1.htm

CCF is dedicated to the cause of cancer care and cure and operates from the G. Kuppuswamy Memorial Hospital, rendering counseling, guidance and educational services to cancer patients and their family members.

GLOBAL CANCER CONCERN INDIA

H-16 Green Park Extension
New Delhi 110 016
Tel: 6100407, 6197899
Fax: 6171028
e-mail: gcci@vsnl.com

GCCI provides assistance in timely diagnosis, home care, education of orphans of deceased patients, rehabilitation, hospices for those who have none to bank upon, etc. The services of GCCI are available in Delhi, Mumbai, Kanpur, Gwalior, Mysore, Chandigarh, Bhopal, Ahmedabad and Amritsar.

INDIAN CANCER SOCIETY (ICS)

Q5-A Jangpura Extension
New Delhi 110 014
Tel: 4319572, 6845230
Fax: 4314907
e-mail: incansoc@nda.vsnl.net.in
Website: www.indiancancersocietydelhi.org

Some of the activities of ICS include cancer detection and prevention through mobile cancer detection services and centres, educational programs, financial and emotional support for cancer patients, etc. Apart from this it also provides diagnostic and treatment services through its newly established cancer hospital with well-equipped staff and equipment. Over the years the Society has succeeded in bringing about innovations and improvements in the control of cancer in India. ICS also publishes the Indian Journal of Cancer, (website: netcolony.com/members/ijc), the only Indian journal that gives you the most recent information on cancer treatment in India and abroad. It contains well-researched original articles on cancer therapy to suit Indian conditions and case histories of cancer patients. The on-line edition has the table of contents and a summary of articles.

JEEVAN JYOT CANCER RELIEF AND CARE TRUST
C/o Jain Fast Food
8 Amritwar Building
Senapati Bapat Marg
Lower Parel
Mumbai 400 013
Maharashtra
Tel: 4928599, 4927287
e-mail: pvsavla@yahoo.com
Website: www.jeevanjyot.org
    The organization takes care of cancer patients, provides free medicine and food.

JEEVODAYA PUBLIC CHARITABLE TRUST HOSPICE FOR CANCER PATIENTS
Jeevodaya Hospice for Cancer Patients
1/272 (old 86) Kamaraj Road
Mathur Manali
P O 600068
Tamil Nadu
Tel: 5555565, 5559671
e-mail: jeevodaya@vsnl.com
Website: www.jeevodaya.org
    Jeevodaya is a professionally manned hospice rendering free palliative care to patients with advanced cancer. The hospice is run under the aegis of the Jeevodaya Public Charitable Trust which is a non-profit organization. It is situated in the serene surroundings of Mathur village, a suburban village on the outskirts of Chennai.

LEUKEMIA RESOURCES CENTER INDIA
Mumbai
Maharashtra
Website: www.leukemiaindia.com

This is an online guide to leukemia related information, services and organizations. The Resources Center helps patients get the information needed to understand available options, make informed decisions, and effectively take charge of living with leukemia.

PAIN AND PALLIATIVE CARE (PPC)
Dept. of Anaesthesiology
KIMS
Hubli 580 022
Karnataka
Tel: 372222, 373853

PPC provides various services to cancer patients as well as emotional support to the family.

V CARE FOUNDATION
132 Maker Tower 'A'
Cuffe Parade
Mumbai 400 005
Maharashtra
Tel: 2188828, 2184457
Fax: 2184457
Website: www.vcare.orchidwebs.com

V Care provides free support, hope and encouragement to patients and their families.

7. USEFUL READING

A Cancer Battle Plan by Anne E Frahm with David J Frahm; published by Jeremy P Tarcher/Putnam, a member of Penguin Putnam Inc., New York, USA

Beating Cancer with Nutrition by Patrick Quillin with Noreen Quillin; published by Nutrition Times Pres Inc., Tulsa, Okalhama, USA

Boundless Energy: The Complete Mind-Body Program for Overcoming Fatigue by Deepak Chopra; published by Rider, an imprint of Ebury Press, Random House, London, UK

Buddha in Daily Life by Richard Causton; published by Rider, an imprint of Ebury Press, Random House, London, UK

Cancer Made Me by Kasthuri Sreenivasan; published by Bharatiya Vidya Bhavan, Bombay, India

Cancer Talk by Selma R Schimmel with Barry Fox; published by Broadway Books, a division of Random House, Inc. New York, USA

Celebration of the Cells: Letters from a Cancer Survivor by R M Lala; published in Viking by Penguin Books India (P) Ltd., New Delhi, India

Chemotherapy & You: A Guide to Self-help During Treatment. Produced by National Cancer Institute, Maryland, USA.

Courage and Contentment by Gurumayi Chidvilasananda. Published by SYDA Foundation, New York, USA.

Creating Health by Deepak Chopra. Published by Thorsons, an imprint of Harper Collins Publishers, London, UK

Cultivating a Daily Meditation by Tenzin Gyatso. Published by the Library of Tibetan Works and Archives, Dharamsala, India

Defeat the Dragon: Cure of Dreaded Diseases with Acupressure by Devendra Vora. Published by Navneet Publications (India) Limited, Mumbai, India.

Eating Hints. Produced by National Cancer Institute, Maryland, USA.

Foods that Heal: The Natural Way to Good Health by H K Bakhru. Published by Orient Paperbacks, a division of Vision Books Pvt. Ltd., Delhi, India.

Getting Well Again by O Carl Simonton, Stephanie Mathews-Simonton and James L Creighton. Published by Bantam Books, a division of Bantam Doubleday, Dell Publishing Group Inc, New York, USA

Heal Your Body by Lousie L Hay; published by Full Circle Publishing, New Delhi, India

Healing Emotions: Conversations with the Dalai Lama on Mindfulness, Emotions and Health. Edited by Daniel Goleman; published by Shambhala Publications, Inc., Boston, USA

Health Through Balance: An Introduction to Tibetan Medicine by Dr. Yeshi Donden; edited and translated by

Jeffery Hopkins; published by Motilal Banarsidass Publishers Private Limited, Delhi, India

Our Daily Bread by Dr William Scott; published by India Bible Literature for RBC Ministries, Chennai, India

Principles of Ayurveda by Anne Green; published by Thorsons, an imprint of Harper Collins Publishers, London, UK

Quantum Healing: Exploring the Frontiers of Mind/Body Medicine by Deepak Chopra; published by Bantam Books, a division of Bantam Doubleday, Dell Publishing Group Inc, New York, USA

Six Months to Live: Learning from a Young Man with Cancer by Daniel Hallock; published by The Plough Publishing House of The Bruderhof Foundation, Sussex, UK

Taking Time; prepared by the Office of Cancer Communications, National Cancer Institute, Maryland, USA

The Beginner's Guide to Zen Buddhism by Jean Smith; published by Bell Tower, a member of the Crown Publishing Group, Random House, Inc., New York, USA

The Healing Family: The Simonton Approach for Families Facing Illness by Stephanie Mathews-Simonton; published by Bantam Books, a division of Transworld Publishers Limited, London, UK

The Joy of Loving: A Guide to Daily Living with Mother Teresa. Compiled by Jaya Chaliha and Edward Le Joly; published in Viking by Penguin Books India (P) Ltd., New Delhi, India

The Joy of Reiki by Nalin Nirula and Renoo Nirula; published by Full Circle Publishing, New Delhi, India

The Path to Tranquility: Daily Meditations; edited by Renuka Singh. Published in Viking by Penguin Books India (P) Ltd., New Delhi, India

The Tibetan Book of Living and Dying by Sogyal Rinpoche; published by Rider, an imprint of The Random House Group Limited, London, UK

Understanding Cancer of the Lung; produced by the Queensland Cancer Fund, Australia

Understanding Emotions; produced by the National Cancer Institute, Maryland, USA

Understanding Nutrition; produced by the Queensland Cancer Fund, Australia

You Can Heal Your Life by Louise L Hay; published by Full Circle Publishing, New Delhi, India

8. IMPORTANT WEBSITES

A simple search on cancer using a search engine like www.google.com leads to nearly 11 million sites on the subject. Getting the basic information is only the first step, but it is an important prerequisite to an in-depth understanding of the disease. If you are just getting started with finding out about cancer, the internet is your best option. Some of the more important and useful websites on the subject are listed below:

www.acor.org

This website hosted by the Association of Cancer Online Resources (ACOR) is a unique collection of online communities designed to provide timely and accurate information in a supportive environment. It offers access to 131 mailing lists that provide support, information, and community to those affected by cancer and related disorders.

www.cancer.org

The website of the American Cancer Society is focused on research and education, patient and community services and a number of patient-based programs.

www.cancercareinc.org

Cancer Care Inc, a national organization in America,

provides patient and family counseling, educational programs, teleconferences and support referrals.

www.cancerguide.org

This website has been created by Steve Dunn, a cancer survivor, and provides basic information on cancer. The website covers individual experiences and a collection of articles on subjects including medical literature, clinical trials, cancer statistics, etc.

www.cancerhopenetwork.org

Cancer Hope Network, USA, provides free confidential support to cancer patients and their families. It matches patients and/or family members with trained volunteers who have undergone similar experiences and treatment.

www.mskcc.org

The website of the Sloane Kettering Memorial provides information on cancer treatment and latest research information, articles and literature.

www.nccf.org

The National Childhood Cancer Foundation, USA, supports and sponsors research and treatment for childhood cancers in top pediatric institutions.

www.ncinih.gov

A program of the National Institute of Health, USA, coordinating a national research program on cancer causes and prevention, detection, diagnosis and treatment.

www.oncolink.upenn.edu

A comprehensive cancer information website from the University of Pennsylvania Cancer Centre. The website contains information regarding specific cancer sites, treatment and emotional support as well as current articles, literature and research information.

A listing of some websites on specific cancers is given below.

BREAST CANCER

www.breastcancer.about.com

This website provides basic information on breast cancer through a series of articles, forums and a regular newsletter. It also has a chat room for discussion and dialogue with other patients.

www.nabco.org

The National Association of Breast Cancer Organizations, USA, provides information and assistance to patients and family members.

www.ntlbcc.org

The National Breast Cancer Coalition, USA, is a grassroot organization that focuses on public education and advocacy for breast cancer awareness.

BRAIN CANCER

www.abta.org

The American Brain Tumor Association provides educational materials, referrals to treatment facilities, support groups and research.

CERVICAL

www.cervicalheath.org

The Centre for Cervical Health provides information on pap tests, useful information and resources.

www.vulvarpainfoundation.org

The Vulvar Pain Foundation provides information on treatment, support and research. It also promotes public awareness.

LEUKEMIA
www.leukemia.org
The Leukemia Society of America, a voluntary health organization, provides counseling and literature.

LUNG CANCER
www.alcase.org
The Alliance for Lung Cancer Advocacy, Support and Education assists lung cancer patients and their families by providing rehabilitation programs and exercises.

www.lungusa.org
The American Lung Association provides cancer information, education, smoking cessation programs and a speaker's bureau.

PROSTATE CANCER
www.afud.org
The American Foundation for Urologic Disease provides research, education, support groups and public awareness for men with prostate cancer.

www.capcure.org
The Association for the Cure of Cancer of the Prostate is a charitable organization that funds research on prostate cancer cure.

9. GLOSSARY OF CANCER TERMINOLOGY

A

Adenocarcinoma: See Carcinoma.

Adenoma: A benign tumor made up of glandular tissue. For example, an adenoma of the pituitary gland may cause it to produce abnormal amounts of hormones.

Adjuvant treatment: Treatment that is added to increase the effectiveness of a primary therapy.

AFP (Alpha fetoprotein): A tumor marker.

Alopecia: The loss of hair, which may include all body hair as well as scalp hair.

Anemia: A condition in which a decreased number of red blood cells may cause symptoms including tiredness, shortness of breath, and weakness.

Anorexia: The loss of appetite.

Antibody: A substance formed by the body to help defend it against infection.

Antiemetic agent: A drug that prevents or controls nausea and vomiting.

Antifungal agent: A drug used to treat fungal infections.

Antigen: Any substance that causes the body to produce natural antibodies.

Antineoplastic agent: A drug that prevents, kills, or blocks the growth and spread of cancer cells.

Arrhythmia: An irregular heartbeat.

Aspiration: The process of removing fluid or tissue, or both, from a specific area.

Asymptomatic: Without the obvious signs or symptoms of the disease.

Autoimmunity: A condition in which the body's immune system mistakenly fights and rejects the body's own tissues.

Axilla: The armpit.

Axillary nodes: Lymph nodes, also called lymph glands, found in the armpit (axilla).

B

Barium enema: The use of a milky solution (barium sulphate) given by an enema to allow x-ray examination of the lower intestinal tract.

Benign growth: A swelling or growth that is not cancerous and does not spread from one part of the body to another.

Biopsy: The surgical removal of tissue for microscopic examination to aid in diagnosis.

Blood count: The number of red blood cells, white blood cells, and platelets in a sample of blood.

Bone marrow: The spongy material found inside the bones. Most blood cells are made in the bone marrow.

Bone marrow biopsy and aspiration: The procedure by which a needle is inserted into a bone to withdraw a sample of bone marrow.

Bone marrow suppression: A decrease in the production of blood cells.

Bone marrow transplant: The infusion of bone marrow into a patient who has been treated with high dose chemotherapy or radiation therapy. Allogeneic: The infusion of bone marrow from one individual (donor) to another. Autologous: The infusion of a patient's own bone marrow previously removed and stored. Syngeneic: The infusion of bone marrow from one identical twin into another.

Bone scan: A picture of the bones using a radioactive dye that shows any injury, disease, or healing. This is a valuable test to determine if cancer has spread to the bone, if anti-cancer therapy has been successful, and if affected bone areas are healing.

Bronchoscopy: The insertion of a flexible, lighted tube through the mouth into the lungs to examine the lungs and airways.

C

Candidiasis: A common fungal infection.

Carcinogen: A substance that causes cancer. For example, nicotine in cigarettes is a carcinogen that causes lung cancer.

Carcinoma: A type of cancer that starts in the skin or the lining of organs. Adenocarcinoma: A malignant tumor arising from glandular tissue. Basal cell carcinoma: The most common type of skin cancer. Bronchogenic carcinoma: A cancer originating in the lungs or airways. Cervical carcinoma: A cancer of the cervix (the neck of the uterus). Endometrial carcinoma: A cancer of the lining of the uterus. Squamous cell carcinoma: Cancer arising from the skin or the surfaces of other structures, such as the mouth, cervix, or lungs.

Cardiomegaly: Enlargement of the heart.

CAT scan (CT scan): A test using computers and x-rays to create images of various parts of the body.

Central venous catheter: A special intravenous tubing that is surgically inserted into a large vein near the heart and exits from the chest or abdomen. The catheter allows medications, fluids, or blood products to be given and blood samples to be taken. (Examples of types of central venous catheters are Broviac, Groshong and Hickman.)

Chemotherapy: The treatment of cancer with drugs. Adjuvant chemotherapy: Chemotherapy given to kill any remaining cancer cells, usually after the detectable tumor is removed by surgery or radiotherapy. Combination chemotherapy: The use of more than one drug during cancer treatment.

Colonoscopy: A procedure to look at the colon or large bowel through a lighted, flexible tube.

Colony-stimulating factor (CSF): An injectable substance used to stimulate the bone marrow to produce more cells.

Cyst: An accumulation of fluid or semi-solid material within a sac.

Cystitis: An inflammation of the bladder.

Cytology: Study of cells under a microscope.

D

Dysphagia: Difficulty in swallowing.

Dyspnea: Difficult or painful breathing; shortness of breath.

Dysuria: Difficult or painful urination.

E

Edema: The accumulation of fluid in a part of the body.

Effusion: A collection of fluid in a body cavity, usually between two adjoining tissues. For example, a pleural effusion is the collection of fluid between two layers of the pleura (the lung's covering).

Electrocardiogram (EKG or ECG): A test that takes recordings of the electrical activity of the heart.

Endoscopy: A procedure looking at the inside of body cavities, such as the esophagus (food pipe) or stomach.

Estrogen: A female hormone produced primarily by the ovaries.

Estrogen receptor assay (ER assay): A test that determines if breast cancer is stimulated by the hormone estrogen.

F

Fine-needle aspiration: A procedure in which a needle is inserted, under local anesthesia, to obtain a sample for the evaluation of suspicious tissue.

Fistula: An abnormal opening between two areas of the body.

Frozen section: A technique in which tissue is removed and then quick-frozen and examined under a microscope by a pathologist.

G

Granulocyte: A type of white blood cell that kills bacteria.

Groshong catheter: See Central venous catheter.

Guaiac test: A test that checks for hidden blood in the stool.

H

Hematocrit (Hct): The percentage of red blood cells in the blood. A low hematocrit measurement indicates anemia.

Hematuria: Blood in the urine.

Herpes simplex: The most common virus that causes sores often seen around the mouth, commonly called cold sores.

Herpes zoster: A virus that settles around certain nerves causing blisters, swelling, and pain. This condition is also called shingles.

Hodgkin's disease: A cancer that affects the lymph nodes. See Lymphoma.

Hospice: A concept of supportive care to meet the special needs of patients and family during the terminal stages of illness. The care may be delivered in the home or hospital by a specially trained team of professionals.

I

Immunosuppression: Weakening of the immune system that causes a lowered ability to fight infection and disease.

Immunotherapy: The artificial stimulation of the body's

immune system to treat or fight disease.

Injection: Pushing medication into the body with the use of a syringe and needle. Intramuscular (IM) injection: Into the muscle. Intravenous (IV) injection: Into the vein. Subcutaneous injection: Into the fatty tissue under the skin.

L

Laryngectomy: The surgical removal of the larynx.

Lesion: A lump or abscess that may be caused by injury or disease such as cancer.

Leukemia: Cancer of the blood. White blood cells may be produced in excessive amounts and are unable to work properly.

Leukocyte: See White blood cells.

Leukopenia: A low number of white blood cells.

Lymphatic system: A network that includes lymph nodes, lymph, and lymph vessels that serves as a filtering system for the blood.

Lymph nodes: Hundreds of small oval bodies that contain lymph. Lymph nodes act as our first line of defense against infections and cancer.

Lymphocytes: White blood cells that kill viruses and defend against the invasion of foreign material.

Lymphoma: A cancer of the lymphatic system. Doctors differentiate between the different lymphomas by the type of cell that is involved in the make-up of the tumor. Treatments depend on the type of cell that is seen.

M

Malignant tumor: A tumor made up of cancer cells of the type that can spread to other parts of the body.

Mammogram (Mammography): A low-dose x-ray of the breasts to determine whether abnormal growths or cysts are present.

Mastectomy: The surgical removal of the breast. Mastectomy-Segmental (lumpectomy): Removal of the lump and a small amount of surrounding breast tissue. Mastectomy-Simple (modified mastectomy): Removal of the entire breast. Mastectomy-Radical: Removal of the entire breast along with underlying muscle and lymph nodes of the armpit.

Melanoma: A cancer of the pigment-forming cells of the skin or the retina of the eye.

Metastasize: To spread from the first cancer site, for example, breast cancer that spreads to the bone.

MRI (Magnetic resonance imaging): A sophisticated test that provides in-depth images of organs and structures in the body.

Mucosa (Mucous membranes): The lining of the mouth and gastrointestinal tract.

Mucositis: Inflammation of the lining of the mouth or gastrointestinal tract.

Myelogram: A x-ray procedure by which a dye is injected into the spinal column to show the pathology of the spinal cord.

Myeloma: A malignant tumor of the bone marrow associated with the production of abnormal proteins.

N

Neoplasm: A new growth of tissue or cells; a tumor that is generally malignant.

Neutropenia: A decreased number of neutrophils, a type of white blood cell.

Non-Hodgkin's lymphoma: A cancer of the lymphatic system. Non-Hodgkin's lymphoma is related to Hodgkin's disease but is made up of different cell types. See Lymphoma.

O

Oncogene: Certain stretches of cellular DNA. Genes that when inappropriately activated, contribute to the malignant transformation of a cell.

Oncologist: A doctor who specializes in oncology.

Oncology: The study and treatment of cancer.

P

Palliative treatment: Treatment aimed at the relief of pain and symptoms of disease but not intended to cure the disease.

Palpation: A procedure using the hands to examine organs such as the breast or prostate.

Pap (Papanicolaou) smear: A test to detect cancer of the cervix.

Pathology: The study of disease by the examination of tissues and body fluids under the microscope. A doctor who specializes in pathology is called a pathologist.

Photosensitivity: Extreme sensitivity to the sun, leaving the patient prone to sunburn. This can be a side effect of some cancer drugs and radiation.

Placebo: An inert substance often used in clinical trials for comparison.

Platelet (Plt): Cells in the blood that are responsible for clotting.

Platelet count: The number of platelets in a blood sample.

Polyp: A growth of tissue protruding into a body cavity, such as a nasal or rectal polyp. Polyps may be benign or malignant.

Port-Implanted: A catheter connected to a quarter-sized disc that is surgically placed just below the skin in the chest or abdomen. The tube is inserted into a large vein or artery directly into the bloodstream. Fluids, drugs, or blood products can be infused, and blood can be drawn through a needle that is stuck into the disc. Examples: Port-o-cath, Infusaport, Lifeport. Port-Peritoneal: A catheter connected to a quarter-sized disc that is surgically placed in the abdomen. The catheter is inserted to deliver chemotherapy to the peritoneum (abdominal cavity).

Primary tumor: The original cancer site. For example, breast cancer that has spread to the bone is still called breast cancer.

Prognosis: The projected outcome of a disease; the life expectancy.

PSA (Prostate-specific antigen): A marker used to determine prostate disease; it may be benign or malignant.

Prosthesis: Artificial replacement of a missing body part.

Protocol: A treatment plan.

R

Radiation therapy: X-ray treatment that damages or kills cancer cells.

Radiologist: A doctor who specializes in the use of x-rays to diagnose and treat disease.

Red blood cells (Erythrocytes): Cells in the blood that deliver oxygen to tissues and take carbon-dioxide from them.

Red blood count (RBC): The number of red blood cells seen in a blood sample.

Regression: The shrinkage of cancer growth.

Relapse: The reappearance of a disease after its apparent cessation.

Remission: Complete or partial disappearance of the signs and symptoms of disease.

S

Sarcoma: A malignant tumor of muscles or connective tissue such as bone and cartilage. Chondrosarcoma: A malignant tumor of cartilage that usually occurs near the ends of the long bones. Ewing's sarcoma: A malignant tumor starting in the bone, affecting the bones of the extremities. It often appears before the age of 20.

Sputum: Secretion produced by the lungs.

Staging: Determination of the extent of cancer in the body.

Steroids: A type of hormone.

T

Tissue: A collection of similar cells. There are four basic types of tissues in the body: epithelial, connective, muscle and nerve.

Tracheostomy: A surgical opening through the trachea in the neck to provide an artificial airway.

Tumor: An abnormal overgrowth of cells. Tumors can be either benign or malignant.

U

Ultrasound examination: The use of high frequency sound waves to aid in diagnosis.

V

Vaccine: A substance injected into the body to stimulate resistance to a specific disease.

Virus: A tiny infectious agent that is smaller than bacteria.

W

White blood cells (WBC): General term for a variety of cells responsible for fighting germs, infection, and allergy-causing agents. Specific white blood cells include granulocytes and lymphocytes.

White blood count (WBC): The actual number of white blood cells seen in a blood sample.

X

X-ray: High-energy electromagnetic radiation used to diagnose disease.